# S C I

# Structured Clinical Interview

# *Manual*

*By* EUGENE I. BURDOCK, Ph.D.

*and* ANNE S. HARDESTY, Ph.D.

*Biometric Laboratory, Department of Psychiatry and Neurology*
*School of Medicine, New York University Medical Center*

Springer Science+Business Media, LLC

Development of this instrument was supported in part
by Public Health Service Research Grant No. 11117
from the National Institute of Mental Health.

Library of Congress Catalog Card Number: 74-78914

ISBN 978-3-662-39357-4      ISBN 978-3-662-40407-2 (eBook)
DOI 10.1007/978-3-662-40407-2

# Preface

The STRUCTURED CLINICAL INTERVIEW (SCI) is the fruit of an eight-year period of development. The idea arose after the *Ward Behavior Inventory* (earlier the *Ward Behavior Rating Scale*) had been constructed. It seemed useful to supplement the description of pathological behavior observed naturalistically on the ward with a technique that would test the readiness of a subject to disclose psychopathology through his discourse in the context of an interview. At first a few questions were constructed to stimulate the production of verbal output for a supplement to the *Ward Behavior Inventory*. These questions were put to the patient by the psychologist after general observation of behavior had been completed by ward personnel. However, it soon became clear that a separate instrument would have the advantage of providing a uniformly controlled stimulus situation in which to assess the subject's behavior in the two-person social setting of the interview. Such an instrument would serve independently to complement and corroborate the report of ward behavior. Early versions of the *Structured Clinical Interview* were originally titled *Biometric Interview* and, later, *Structured Clinical Interview and Inventory*. By 1963 enough data had been accumulated to determine item frequencies, to cluster items into rational subgroups and to test reliability and validity. The present edition of the SCI was essentially completed by 1965 but certain small refinements in format were made as recently as 1968.

Many individuals contributed to the shaping of the *Structured Clinical Interview* during the eight-year period of its development. The authors would like to express their appreciation to the individual interviewers, to the data processors, and to the institutional directors who expedited the accumulation of the data reported here, as well as to the subjects, all of whom enriched the project and increased our understanding of psychopathology.

A complete listing of those to whom we are obligated is not possible, but several individuals must be singled out because of longterm and especially meaningful contributions to this endeavor.

Most of this work was accomplished while the authors were on the staff of Biometrics Research at the New York State Psychiatric Institute. Our special thanks is expressed to Dr. Joseph Zubin, Chief of Biometrics Research, New York State Department of Mental Hygiene, for his interest and support, and to Dr. Lawrence C. Kolb, Director of the New York State Psychiatric Institute, for his facilitation of the necessary research. Dr. Samuel Gershon, Director Neuropsychopharmacology Research Unit, New York University School of Medicine, contributed significantly to the validation studies by pitting psychiatric judgment against the sensitivity of the instrument in drug research.

3

Mr. Victor Bergenn served with distinction for several years in helping to control the logistics of data collection as well as in supervising in the field. Mrs. Marylin Wechselblatt's competence was unexcelled in data collection and data analysis. Dr. Joseph Fleiss and Mrs. Bu Young Chang provided exceptional help in statistics and programming.

A particular debt of gratitude is due Mrs. Matilda Baker for her infinite good humor and patience, and the skill with which she prepared what seemed the infinity of revisions which preceded the final version of the SCI.

*New York City*　　　　　　　　　　　　　　　　　　　　　　　E.I.B.
*June, 1969*　　　　　　　　　　　　　　　　　　　　　　　　A.S.H.

## CONTENTS

# S C I

## Structured Clinical Interview

### PURPOSE AND DESCRIPTION

The STRUCTURED CLINICAL INTERVIEW (SCI) is a psychological technique for the detection and assessment of psychopathology. Its effective application requires an examiner who can combine the experimental with the clinical attitude. It is thus a tool for the pychologist because his training uniquely qualifies him for this role. Some supervised experience with the technique is of course necessary to assure common standards of judgment.

The SCI provides a standardized psychological method for the evaluation of psychopathology comparable to the standardized psychological methods used for the evaluation of intelligence. Such an evaluation, derived from accumulated clinical knowledge, has to be based on a representative sample of critical behaviors and attitudes that can be reliably assessed in an individual testing session, that are discriminating, and that are amenable to quantitative treatment. The resultant scores, when standardized against appropriate norms, can be used for individual assessment, for comparisons between groups and between individuals, and for determining changes in individuals or groups over the course of time or in response to treatment. Although SCI scores and profiles will often serve as adjuncts to diagnosis, it must be emphasized that the SCI is a psychological, not a psychiatric, technique; it involves a carefully controlled stimulus situation, not a free inquiry; it is ahistorical; it focuses on manifest behavior; and it is not couched in psychiatric terminology.

The SCI consists of both an interview protocol and an inventory of 179 behavioral items. The examiner records his judgments of the psychological significance of the subject's responses by checking YES or NO for each of the items as the interview progresses. The interview usually takes about 20 to 30 minutes. Since the examiner records his judgments during the interview, no additional time is required for completion of the schedule after the subject has departed.

The SCI is intended both for screening and for determination of changes in psychopathology. Its design combines features derived from five sources: (1) the individual psychological test, (2) the survey interview, (3) the projective techniques, (4) the personality questionnaire, and (5) the rating scale.

5

1. The individual test can be viewed as a miniature psychological experiment in which the examiner manipulates certain independent stimulus variables, at the same time trying to exclude extraneous stimuli. The responses of the subject can then be analyzed as the dependent variable. The method seeks to introduce into the face-to-face clinical setting some of the control and rigor of the psychological laboratory. The relation between the amount of control and the quantity of reliable information obtained is curvilinear. Up to a point, as rigor is increased, the quality of the clinical information obtained is also increased. However, a point of diminishing returns is eventually reached beyond which the clinically significant information dwindles. In some interview studies of mental patients so many constraints have been imposed on the subjects that their output has been reduced to verbal behavior denuded of clinical detail.

2. The survey interview is widely used in social psychology and is the method of choice in sociology and political science for sampling opinions and attitudes. The survey has the virtue of providing current information elicited at the subject's convenience, either in his home or in a public place. The essential ingredients for reliable results are an adequate sampling design, a properly constructed protocol, and trained and motivated interviewers. Surveys of mental illness frequently founder because the protocol is too gross and the field interviewers are inadequately trained.

3. The projective techniques provide plausible contexts in which the subject is likely to display aspects of his personality that would be shielded from direct inquiry. However, these techniques are refractory to standardization, the stimulus material being too loosely structured to assure comparability from subject to subject and occasion to occasion, while the criteria against which the responses are assessed are of such subtlety that the same response may be rated positive or negative in accordance with variable dynamic inferences.

4. The personality questionnaire has the virtue of providing a quantitative, objective record of the subject's self-evaluation. But deficiencies in insight, as well as lack of an opportunity to qualify the responses may bias the results in an unknown way. Landis and Katz (1934) studied response sets on the personality questionnaire by interviewing subjects after they had completed a questionnaire. They found that any of the three alternative choices to one of the questions could be the result of the same response set.

5. Rating scales are, for one thing, excellent training devices because they require a systematic scrutiny of all the relevant behaviors. Beginning observers and interviewers often are at a loss as to what they should observe. A rating scale alerts them to what they should look for. When used by experienced observers, rating scales provide objective quantifiable judgments for both scientific and administrative purposes. The most effective rating scales are those which focus on observable behavior. However, rating scales are usually employed without control of the stimulus context from which the observations

are drawn, a defect which compromises comparability; and they commonly have the additional defect of depending on retrospective evaluations, with all the attendant errors of recall that retrospection is heir to.

The SCI requires the examiner to set down his judgments of the behavior of the subject during the course of the examination, as in such individual tests as the WAIS and the Stanford-Binet. The tone of inquiry is relatively mild, with stimulus questions which focus on specific content areas relevant for evaluation of psychopathology but that do not insist on detailed disclosures, thus avoiding the effect of pressure. The inquiry is open-ended and somewhat ambiguous, making it necessary for the subject to work out his responses, which thus tend to reflect his own rather than the examiner's ideas. The items are arranged in the order in which the corresponding behaviors are most likely to be elicited by the stimulus inquiries, so that the examiner can complete the schedule during the interview, a technique which retains the quantitative feature of the questionnaire as well as its immediacy but which reflects a professional judgment rather than a self-evaluation. The procedure strikes an effective compromise between detail and brevity, so as to be suitable for screening in a wide variety of situations. A concentration on current status rather than on historical or dynamic source material makes possible repeated applications for assessment of changes in pathology over time.

The comparatively neutral stimuli used in the SCI are intended to minimize any tendency of the subject toward acquiescence or disavowal. It is, therefore, desirable that the SCI be administered before any more probing inquiries, so as to avoid possible after-effects of reinforcement of such response tendencies.

The inventory was constructed by identifying in the psychological and psychiatric literature areas of psychopathology generally recognized as having symptom significance. From each of these areas were drawn representative verbalizations, attitudes, and actions significant of psychopathology. These behaviors were then broken down into discrete items. The interview in turn was constructed so as to provide a uniform stimulus context in which to direct the subject's attention toward these areas of adaptation and to give him an opportunity to exhibit ideation and behavior from which the psychologist can judge the presence or absence of psychopathology. The approach to areas of potential pathology is oblique rather than direct, the interviewer's inquiries being so phrased as to offer the subject the opportunity to invest them with his own meanings. Such direct questions as are necessary are cast in a form to preclude simple "yes" or "no" responses. Although the stimuli are ambiguous, the responses are evaluated with explicit reference to the preselected behavioral items of the schedule.

While the ordering of the items facilitates the examiner's task of locating relevant behaviors, he needs to be alert to record a significant item when it occurs earlier or later in the interview.

7

The inventory is molecular, with items so worded that a judgment of "YES" by the examiner indicates presence of an element of maladaptive behavior. The items of the SCI have been clustered into the following ten nonoverlapping subtests:

1. Anger-Hostility (reflected either in verbalization or in behavior)—27 items: fit of anger; trouble with the law; irritable; jealous; bitterly envious; feels hatred for relative or associate; is angry when criticized; people push him around; does not care if he harms others; hits or attacks people; expresses resentment; accuses interviewer; acts contemptuous; is belligerent; shouts, yells; menacing gesture; throws something; bangs or stamps; tears or breaks; looks angry; turns away.

2. Conceptual Dysfunction (disturbances of concept formation, concept retention, or concept evocation which interfere with cognitive functioning, and which express themselves in defects of communication, orientation, memory, attention, and concentration)—28 items: fails to give name, date, place; assumes false role; does not remember how he came; gives implausible or incomplete account; difficulty in recall; tells of fit, seizure; does not recognize evidence of disturbance; misidentifies; obscure or cryptic explanations; mechanical repetitions; gibberish; aimless talk; minute elaborations; contradictory explanations; forgets what he is talking about; distractable; becomes preoccupied; pressure of speech; blurred speech, inaudible or incoherent.

3. Fear-Worry (reports or displays of apprehensiveness, nervousness, or anxiousness)—12 items: bothered by feelings of nervousness or anxiety; has periods of depression; worries a lot or cannot stop; has lots of fears or fears of different things; has fear of insanity or of losing control; has irrational fear; is concerned about panic; is depressed or despondent; broods; has irrelevant thoughts; sense of humor lost; weeps.

4. Incongruous Behavior (modes of expression which seem contradictory to one another or which are anomalous and unusual ways of doing usual things) —25 items: drags feet; hands are clammy; face dirty; hair unkempt; dirty or bizarre clothes; smells of urine or feces; tells of compulsive acts; incongruous emotional response; gesticulates; frenzied excitement; fleeting expressions; frightened expression; attack of panic; stands up; rubs, scratches, picks; pulls or tugs; rituals; writhes; restless; poses; tic; fidgets; giggles; belches, clucks, grunts; tremor.

5. Incongruous Ideation (contradictory emotions, strange or bizarre notions incompatible with reality, outright delusions, or ideas which are uncoupled from the socially expected emotional toning, i.e., ideation with inappropriate affect or without affect)—28 items: blames others; tells of period of elation; nothing bothers him; enjoys cruelty; "possessed"; enjoys tragic events; says he feels "high"; has uncorroborated disease; body

changing in size or shape; body rotting; has fatal illness or is about to die; people or things look weird or distorted; food suspicious or poisoned; weird thoughts; things unreal or dreamlike; being punished for sin; harmed by stranger; mistreated by authority; ideas of reference; harassed or persecuted; mind controlled; has unknown enemy; superhuman power or knowledge; world wide fame; idée fixe; expresses extreme elation.

6. Lethargy-Dejection (reflected in physical as well as in emotional expression)—17 items: feels tired; does not smile; no interests; enjoys nothing; no plans; flat affect; says little; faint voice; monotone; slow speech; sad expression or dejected posture; sighs; immobile; eyes closed or head averted; impassive expression; slow movements; hardly talks.

7. Perceptual Dysfunction (hallucinatory experiences)—6 items: visual hallucinations; micropsia or macropsia; auditory hallucinations; tactile hallucinations; olfactory hallucinations; somatic hallucinations.

8. Physical Complaints (reports of somatic problems)—17 items: motor or sensory dysfunction; dissatisfied with size or strength; palpitations, faintness, dizziness; anorexia.

9. Self Depreciation (feelings of guilt, inferiority or worthlessness)—20 items: feelings dried up; alcoholic or drug addict; rash; difficulty in decision making; afraid of acting out; getting nowhere; dissatisfied with appearance; suicidal thoughts; suicidal intentions; masochistic; impaired memory; wishful thinking; people avoid him; feels distant from people; no friends; guilt feelings; inferiority feelings; negative attitude toward future; intense regret.

10. Sexual Problems (difficulties stemming from sexual attitudes or behavior)—9 items: uncomfortable when asked about opposite sex; has difficulty with opposite sex; impotent or frigid; sexual habits get him into trouble; worried about masturbation; homosexual; nymphomaniac; exposes genitals; sexual suggestion; sexual advance.

9

# DEVELOPMENT AND APPLICATIONS

## INTERNAL CONSISTENCY

In the first applications of the S.C.I. the observed items of maladaptive behavior were simply summed to provide a measure of level of pathology.

Table 1. Composition and Reliability of Subtests of the *Structured Clinical Interview* on a Sample of 183 Mental Patients

| Subtest I (Anger-Hostility) | | | | Subtest 2 (Conceptual Dysfunction) | | | | Subtest 3 (Fear-Worry) | | | | Subtest 4 (Incongruous Behavior) | | | |
|---|---|---|---|---|---|---|---|---|---|---|---|---|---|---|---|
| Item | Freq. | $r_{pb_1}$ | $r_{pb_T}$ | Item | Freq. | $r_{pb_2}$ | $r_{pb_T}$ | Item | Freq. | $r_{pb_3}$ | $r_{pb_T}$ | Item | Freq. | $r_{pb_4}$ | $r_{pb_T}$ |
| 25 | 7 | .10 | -.02 | 7 | 2 | .19 | .12 | 15 | 68 | .38 | .07 | 1 | 5 | .02 | .07 |
| 27 | 2 | .25 | .14 | 8 | 15 | .47 | .36 | 17 | 54 | .28 | -.15 | 2 | 5 | .21 | .04 |
| 29 | 5 | .11 | .12 | 9 | 16 | .55 | .30 | 20 | 23 | .31 | .08 | 3 | 7 | .15 | .12 |
| 73 | 3 | .17 | .08 | 10 | 2 | .38 | .13 | 21 | 14 | .19 | .01 | 4 | 7 | .11 | .06 |
| 74 | 6 | .27 | .05 | 11 | 3 | .27 | .10 | 22 | 39 | .19 | .15 | 5 | 2 | .17 | .11 |
| 75 | 3 | .20 | .16 | 12 | 18 | .46 | .28 | 23 | 7 | .09 | .02 | 6 | 0 | 0 | 0 |
| 76 | 29 | .29 | .06 | 13 | 44 | .54 | .13 | 24 | 10 | .16 | -.06 | 26 | 1 | -.04 | -.04 |
| 77 | 5 | .35 | .14 | 63 | 15 | .01 | .18 | 37 | 60 | .26 | 0 | 113 | 11 | .18 | .11 |
| 78 | 28 | .45 | .12 | 64 | 8 | .08 | .01 | 66 | 64 | .42 | .26 | 149 | 1 | -.04 | .16 |
| 79 | 22 | .58 | .22 | 110 | 66 | .49 | .12 | 68 | 7 | .13 | .17 | 150 | 1 | .12 | .08 |
| 84 | 6 | .14 | .14 | 116 | 19 | .10 | .06 | 71 | 42 | .13 | .17 | 151 | 3 | -.03 | -.03 |
| 93 | 5 | .44 | .16 | 117 | 2 | .38 | .13 | 155 | 23 | .15 | .20 | 156 | 9 | .10 | .19 |
| 96 | 4 | .12 | .23 | 120 | 39 | .33 | .28 | | | | | 157 | 0 | 0 | 0 |
| 97 | 0 | 0 | 0 | 121 | 7 | .32 | .24 | | | | | 160 | 0 | 0 | 0 |
| 101 | 2 | .14 | .10 | 122 | 4 | .19 | .03 | | | | | 161 | 4 | .21 | .11 |
| 114 | 26 | .11 | .14 | 123 | 16 | .39 | .21 | | | | | 163 | 3 | .12 | .07 |
| 115 | 1 | .10 | .12 | 124 | 30 | .09 | .13 | | | | | 164 | 1 | -.04 | .12 |
| 118 | 7 | .10 | .14 | 125 | 11 | .26 | .21 | | | | | 165 | 1 | .20 | -.03 |
| 135 | 13 | .20 | .04 | 129 | 5 | .15 | .19 | | | | | 166 | 3 | .16 | .09 |
| 136 | 1 | .20 | .10 | 130 | 10 | .26 | .09 | | | | | 168 | 1 | .20 | .13 |
| 143 | 0 | 0 | 0 | 131 | 9 | .37 | .25 | | | | | 169 | 3 | .21 | .17 |
| 144 | 0 | 0 | 0 | 132 | 19 | .35 | .16 | | | | | 170 | 18 | .11 | .12 |
| 145 | 0 | 0 | 0 | 133 | 7 | .22 | .22 | | | | | 172 | 7 | .05 | .02 |
| 146 | 0 | 0 | 0 | 138 | 8 | .23 | .17 | | | | | 173 | 1 | .20 | .13 |
| 147 | 7 | .15 | .13 | 140 | 13 | .15 | .09 | | | | | 174 | 5 | .29 | .08 |
| 148 | 0 | 0 | 0 | 141 | 1 | .06 | -.04 | | | | | | | | |
| 159 | 10 | .02 | .19 | 142 | 9 | .34 | .24 | | | | | | | | |
| | | | | 178 | 11 | .28 | .31 | | | | | | | | |

This procedure was supported by studies of the internal consistency of the SCI, a preliminary form of which was reported on at the Eastern Psychological Association in 1962 (Burdock & Hardesty, 1962). Point biserial correlations were computed between each item and total score on a sample of 75 successive admissions to a state research hospital during 1961. Although this sample showed a restricted range of pathology because of the admission policy of the institution at that time, 98 items occurred with sufficient frequency (at least six subjects) to justify consideration of the point biserial.

Table 1 (continued)

Subtest 5 (Incongruous Ideation)

| Item | Freq. | $r_{pb_5}$ | $r_{pb_T}$ |
|---|---|---|---|
| 14 | 22 | .14 | .09 |
| 16 | 2 | .02 | -.02 |
| 19 | 1 | .08 | .04 |
| 28 | 1 | .21 | .16 |
| 31 | 1 | .08 | .13 |
| 35 | 0 | 0 | 0 |
| 36 | 5 | .07 | .05 |
| 43 | 2 | .02 | .07 |
| 45 | 0 | 0 | 0 |
| 46 | 0 | 0 | 0 |
| 47 | 3 | .07 | .02 |
| 51 | 6 | .05 | .10 |
| 56 | 1 | .02 | -.02 |
| 67 | 34 | .48 | .38 |
| 69 | 4 | .07 | -.04 |
| 91 | 0 | 0 | 0 |
| 94 | 10 | .20 | .21 |
| 95 | 6 | .30 | .21 |
| 98 | 8 | .28 | .23 |
| 99 | 8 | .15 | .25 |
| 100 | 2 | -.02 | .05 |
| 102 | 3 | .34 | .22 |
| 103 | 3 | .18 | .10 |
| 109 | 2 | .21 | .03 |
| 126 | 2 | .21 | .13 |
| 127 | 3 | .34 | .22 |
| 128 | 5 | .10 | .15 |
| 152 | 2 | .07 | .01 |

Subtest 6 (Lethargy-Dejection)

| Item | Freq. | $r_{pb_6}$ | $r_{pb_T}$ |
|---|---|---|---|
| 40 | 39 | .20 | .23 |
| 72 | 52 | .46 | .27 |
| 104 | 19 | .50 | .30 |
| 105 | 28 | .55 | .36 |
| 107 | 74 | .24 | .28 |
| 112 | 18 | .16 | .14 |
| 119 | 32 | .19 | -.14 |
| 134 | 13 | .12 | .07 |
| 137 | 16 | .22 | .09 |
| 139 | 8 | .18 | .10 |
| 153 | 55 | .27 | .19 |
| 154 | 14 | .16 | .09 |
| 158 | 5 | .06 | -.12 |
| 162 | 13 | .43 | .27 |
| 171 | 38 | .37 | .16 |
| 175 | 9 | .28 | .11 |
| 179 | 5 | .41 | .13 |

Subtest 7 (Perceptual Dysfunction)

| Item | Freq. | $r_{pb_7}$ | $r_{pb_T}$ |
|---|---|---|---|
| 49 | 6 | .10 | .16 |
| 50 | 0 | 0 | 0 |
| 52 | 13 | .19 | .06 |
| 53 | 6 | .10 | .12 |
| 57 | 4 | .04 | -.02 |
| 70 | 1 | .15 | -.03 |

Subtest 8 (Physical Complaints)

| Item | Freq. | $r_{pb_8}$ | $r_{pb_T}$ |
|---|---|---|---|
| 39 | 22 | .19 | .13 |
| 41 | 25 | .29 | .19 |
| 42 | 8 | .11 | .10 |
| 44 | 10 | .06 | .21 |
| 54 | 25 | .06 | 0 |
| 55 | 46 | .09 | .08 |
| 58 | 7 | .08 | .10 |

Subtest 9 (Self Depreciation)

| Item | Freq. | $r_{pb_9}$ | $r_{pb_T}$ |
|---|---|---|---|
| 18 | 4 | .20 | .11 |
| 30 | 25 | -.08 | -.11 |
| 32 | 2 | -.02 | -.06 |
| 33 | 11 | .29 | .17 |
| 34 | 6 | .19 | .10 |
| 38 | 22 | .20 | .13 |
| 48 | 7 | .22 | .28 |
| 59 | 19 | .18 | .07 |
| 60 | 2 | .07 | .04 |
| 61 | 16 | -.01 | -.05 |
| 62 | 47 | .17 | .22 |
| 65 | 3 | .17 | 0 |
| 80 | 5 | .35 | .16 |
| 81 | 14 | .13 | -.02 |
| 82 | 23 | .19 | .12 |
| 83 | 39 | .07 | .24 |
| 92 | 10 | .03 | -.01 |
| 106 | 26 | .28 | .11 |
| 108 | 28 | .16 | .24 |
| 111 | 27 | .27 | .20 |

Subtest 10 (Sexual Problems)

| Item | Freq. | $r_{pb_{10}}$ | $r_{pb_T}$ |
|---|---|---|---|
| 85 | 21 | .13 | 0 |
| 86 | 19 | .26 | .06 |
| 87 | 10 | .17 | -.04 |
| 88 | 2 | .03 | .13 |
| 89 | 2 | .03 | .01 |
| 90 | 6 | .21 | .01 |
| 167 | 0 | 0 | 0 |
| 176 | 2 | .03 | .02 |
| 177 | 1 | .08 | .01 |

11

Of these, 46 items had 95% confidence limits which excluded zero.

Four criteria were used for assigning items to the subtests: (1) Initially, items were assigned to subtest areas a priori on the basis of clinical and theoretical criteria. (2) Point biserial correlations were then computed between each item and every subtest (with the target item omitted from the subtest). (3) Frequency of occurrence of each item was balanced against magnitude of correlation in order not to exclude rare but apparently critical behaviors. (4) Stability of correlation was determined by replication of the point biserial correlations in samples of chronic resident patients, of new admissions, and of normals.

The authors examined each item in the light of the four criteria, and reassigned items on the basis of discussion and agreement. After several reshufflings of items and recomputations of the point biserials, when no further improvement seemed obtainable, the final assignments of items to the subtests were determined. Table 1 displays the items in each subtest, the point biserial correlations of each item with its subtest and with total, as well as its frequency of occurrence in a sample of 183 hospitalized mental patients. In Table 2 the intercorrelations among the subtests and total are shown for the same sample of 183 mental patients. The relative independence of the subtests from one another is reflected in their low intercorrelations. Correspondingly low intercorrelations were obtained from a sample of 870 hospitalized mental patients in an earlier study (Burdock & Hardesty, 1968).

Table 2. Intercorrelations Among Ten Subtests and Total of the *Structured Clinical Interview* for 183 Mental Hospital Patients

| Subtests | 1 | 2 | 3 | 4 | 5 | 6 | 7 | 8 | 9 | 10 | Total |
|---|---|---|---|---|---|---|---|---|---|---|---|
| 1 | – | .16 | -.11 | .10 | .32 | .09 | .01 | -.01 | .12 | .07 | .43 |
| 2 | | – | -.24 | .27 | .47 | .11 | .11 | .07 | -.06 | -.05 | .56 |
| 3 | | | | 05 | -.04 | .05 | -.03 | .25 | .38 | -.07 | .32 |
| 4 | | | | – | .14 | .01 | .05 | .06 | .03 | .11 | .37 |
| 5 | | | | | – | .09 | .21 | .01 | .01 | .11 | .54 |
| 6 | | | | | | – | .02 | .09 | .13 | -.07 | .52 |
| 7 | | | | | | | – | .13 | .03 | .01 | .20 |
| 8 | | | | | | | | – | .18 | -.09 | .35 |
| 9 | | | | | | | | | – | .15 | .49 |
| 10 | | | | | | | | | | – | .12 |

## DIFFERENTIATION AMONG SUBJECTS

The power of the SCI to differentiate among subjects was tested initially on total scores, i.e., the sums of items significant of pathology. The first of these tests was carried out with an early form of the SCI on a series of successive admissions to a psychiatric research hospital. Simultaneous independent observations were made by four psychologists on 28 patients. In order to obtain multiple simultaneous observations, the interviews were conducted in a special interview room which had an observation booth with a one-way window and stereophonic amplification of sound. The interviewer and each observer independently filled in the inventory as the interview progressed. Table 3 shows the results of a two-way analysis of variance of these data. The intraclass R of .77 indicates that the major part of the variance assigned to the patients can be attributed to actual differences among the subjects (Burdock, Fleiss & Hardesty, 1963). Table 4 lists the results of analyses of a series of studies at different hospitals in which mental patients were rated by two or three observers, one of whom conducted the interview in the presence of the others. Generally, intraclass correlations for total scores have tended to average in the .80's.

Table 3. Analysis of Variance of Total Scores on the *Structured Clinical Interview*

(1961)

| Source | MS | df |
|--------|-----|-----|
| Patients | 99.06 | 27 |
| Observers | 43.39 | 3 |
| Residual | 6.72 | 81 |

$$R_{intraclass} = \frac{s^2_{pt}}{s^2_{pt} + s^2_{res}} = \frac{MS_{pt} - MS_{res}}{MS_{pt} + 3MS_{res}} = .77$$

$$s^2_{obs} = \frac{MS_{obs} - MS_{res}}{N} = 1.31$$

Note--Data are from 28 patients in a psychiatric research hospital rated by 4 observers.

13

Table 4. Intraclass Correlations for Total Scores of the *Structured Clinical Interview*

| Study | N | No. of Observers | $R_{intraclass}$ | $s^2_{res}$ | $s^2_{obs}$ |
|-------|-----|------|------|-------|------|
| P2 | 26 | 3 | .85 | 6.94 | .02 |
| P3 | 15 | 2 | .83 | 12.79 | 0 |
| M1 | 37 | 2 | .92 | 4.48 | 0 |
| M2 | 10 | 2 | .64 | 5.34 | 0 |
| M3 | 25 | 3 | .89 | 9.60 | .75 |
| M4 | 37 | 2 | .80 | 12.09 | 1.03 |
| B2 | 83 | 2 | .83 | 9.87 | 1.65 |

The differentiating potential of the ten subtests of the SCI has been examined in three studies in each of which two judges observed the subjects simultaneously. The subjects of Study I were 25 mental patients who had been in a state hospital over two years. Study II included a number of normals in addition to acute mental patients from two different hospitals. The subjects of Study III were all patients admitted to the psychiatric division of a general hospital. The intraclass correlation coefficients shown in Table 5 reflect some attenuation due to the fact that each of the subtests includes only a fraction of the items.

## OBSERVER AGREEMENT

An index of inter-observer variability can be constructed from the two-way analysis of variance, as shown in Table 3. In this study with an early form of the SCI, analysis of total scores yielded an observer variance of 1.31 for four observers. This value is about one-fifth the magnitude of the residual error variance of 6.72. In the subsequent studies listed in Table 4 observer variance tends to be vanishingly small. For the subtests reported in Table 5, observer variances for paired observers are approximately zero.

## TRANSFORMATION

Figures 1 and 2 show the frequency distributions of total raw scores for two of the samples of community subjects whose scores have provided baselines against which to compare the profiles of mental patients. The first sample drawn from the community consisted of 48 subjects, 40 female, 8 male. Their ages ranged between 19 and 31 years. Twenty-seven of the subjects were students in a medical school course for physical therapists, 12 were graduate students in psychology, and the remaining 9 were young women employed in professional and business occupations. The second

14

Table 5. Summary of Components of Variance for Subtests of the SCI

| Study | Subtests | | | | | | | | | |
|---|---|---|---|---|---|---|---|---|---|---|
| | 1 | 2 | 3 | 4 | 5 | 6 | 7 | 8 | 9 | 10 |
| Intraclass Correlation [a] | | | | | | | | | | |
| I  (N=25) | .66 | .49 | .84 | .34 | .35 | .55 | .77 | .76 | .69 | .93 |
| II  (N=76) | .82 | .85 | .85 | .46 | .77 | .66 | .80 | .78 | .85 | .63 |
| III  (N=38) | .83 | .75 | .69 | .71 | .71 | .78 | .75 | .64 | .67 | .63 |
| Residual Variance [b] | | | | | | | | | | |
| I  (N=25) | .10 | .20 | .06 | .21 | .15 | .08 | .02 | .07 | .11 | .02 |
| II  (N=76) | .07 | .07 | .06 | .15 | .10 | .13 | .04 | .07 | .06 | .08 |
| III  (N=38) | .06 | .09 | .08 | .11 | .10 | .09 | .07 | .11 | .09 | .11 |
| Observer Variance [c] | | | | | | | | | | |
| I  (N=25) | 0 | 0 | .05 | 0 | .01 | .01 | 0 | 0 | .01 | 0 |
| II  (N=76) | 0 | 0 | 0 | 0 | .01 | .01 | 0 | 0 | 0 | 0 |
| III  (N=38) | 0 | 0 | 0 | 0 | 0 | 0 | 0 | 0 | .02 | 0 |

Note--Each study was carried out by a pair of observers, one of whom conducted the interview in the presence of the other.

$$[a] \quad R_{intraclass} = \frac{s^2_{subj}}{s^2_{subj} + s^2_{res}} = \frac{MS_{subj} - MS_{res}}{MS_{subj} + MS_{res}}$$

$$[b] \quad s^2_{res} = MS_{res}$$

$$[c] \quad s^2_{obs} = \frac{MS_{obs} - MS_{res}}{N}$$

sample was composed of 95 referrals to a vocational advisement agency. Their ages ranged from 18 to 56 years. There were 73 males and 22 females. The frequency distributions of both samples resemble exponential decay curves. Figures 3 and 4 give the frequency distributions for two samples of hospitalized mental patients. These distributions are also markedly skewed. In Figures 5 and 6, frequency distributions of total raw scores for two samples of psychiatric outpatients are seen to resemble those of the inpatients.

15

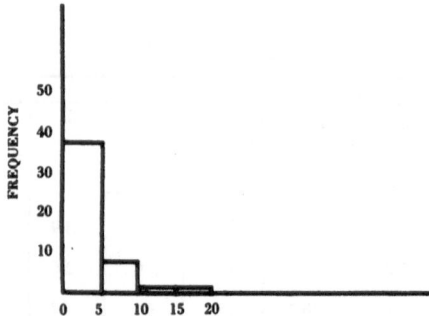

Fig. 1. Frequency distribution of total SCI scores for 48 subjects in the community

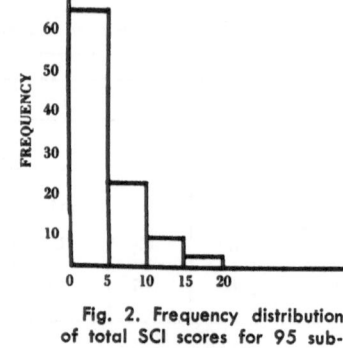

Fig. 2. Frequency distribution of total SCI scores for 95 subjects in the community

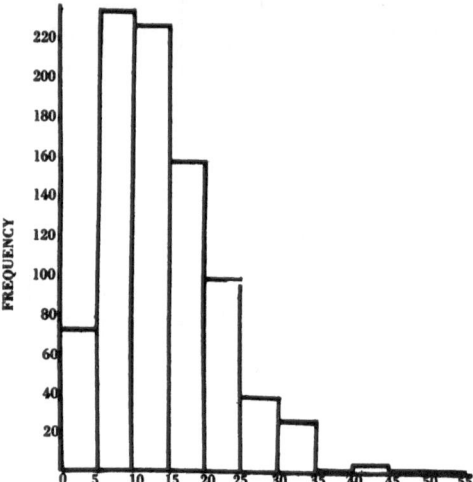

Fig. 3. Frequency distribution of total SCI scores for 870 hospitalized mental patients

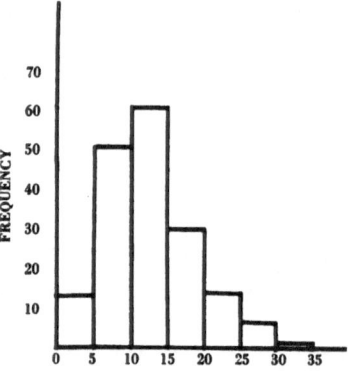

Fig. 4. Frequency distribution of total SCI scores for 183 hospitalized mental patients

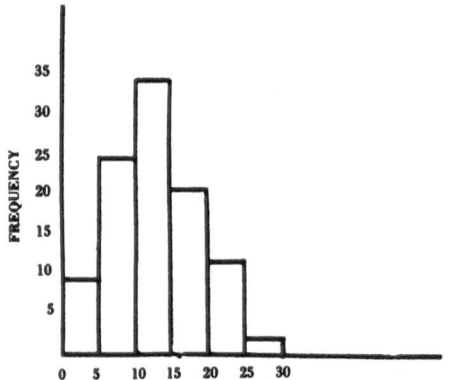

Fig. 5. Frequency distribution of total score for 105 psychiatric outpatients

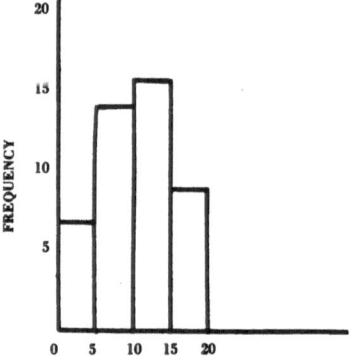

Fig. 6. Frequency distribution of total scores for 46 psychiatric outpatients

16

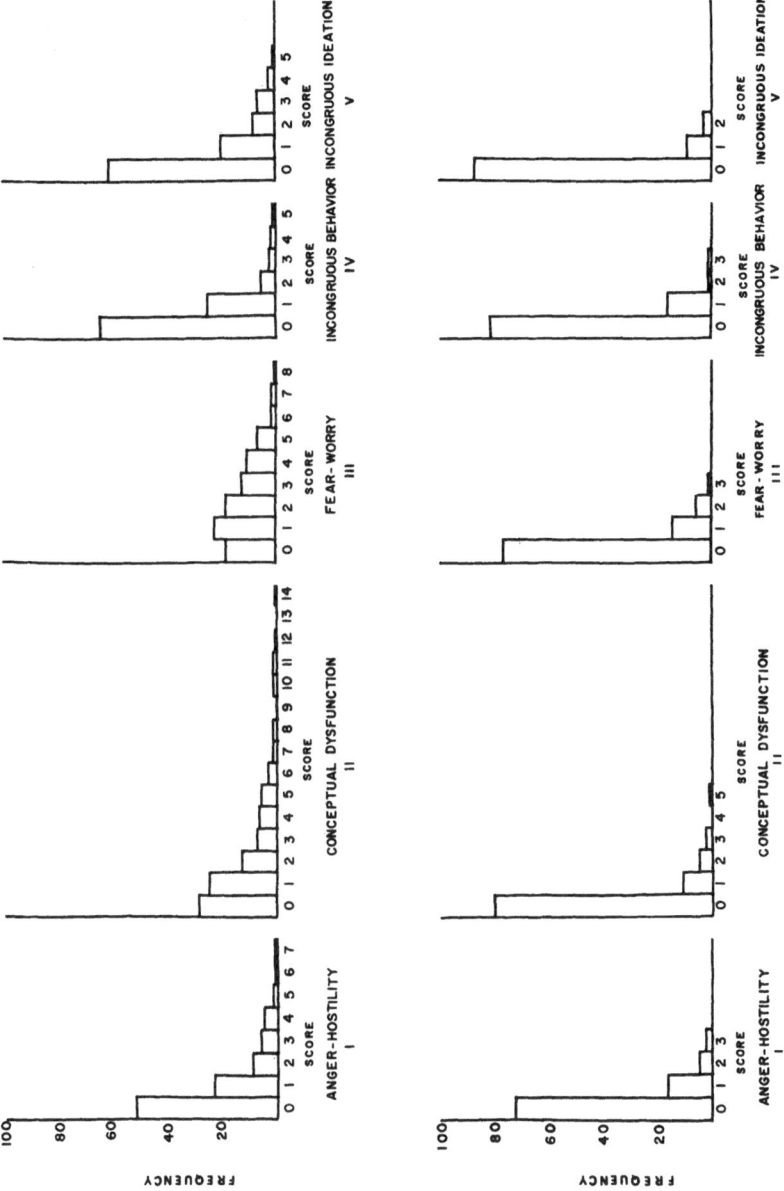

Fig. 7. Frequency distributions of SCI subtest scores of (above) 183 hospitalized mental patients and (below) 95 subjects in the community

17

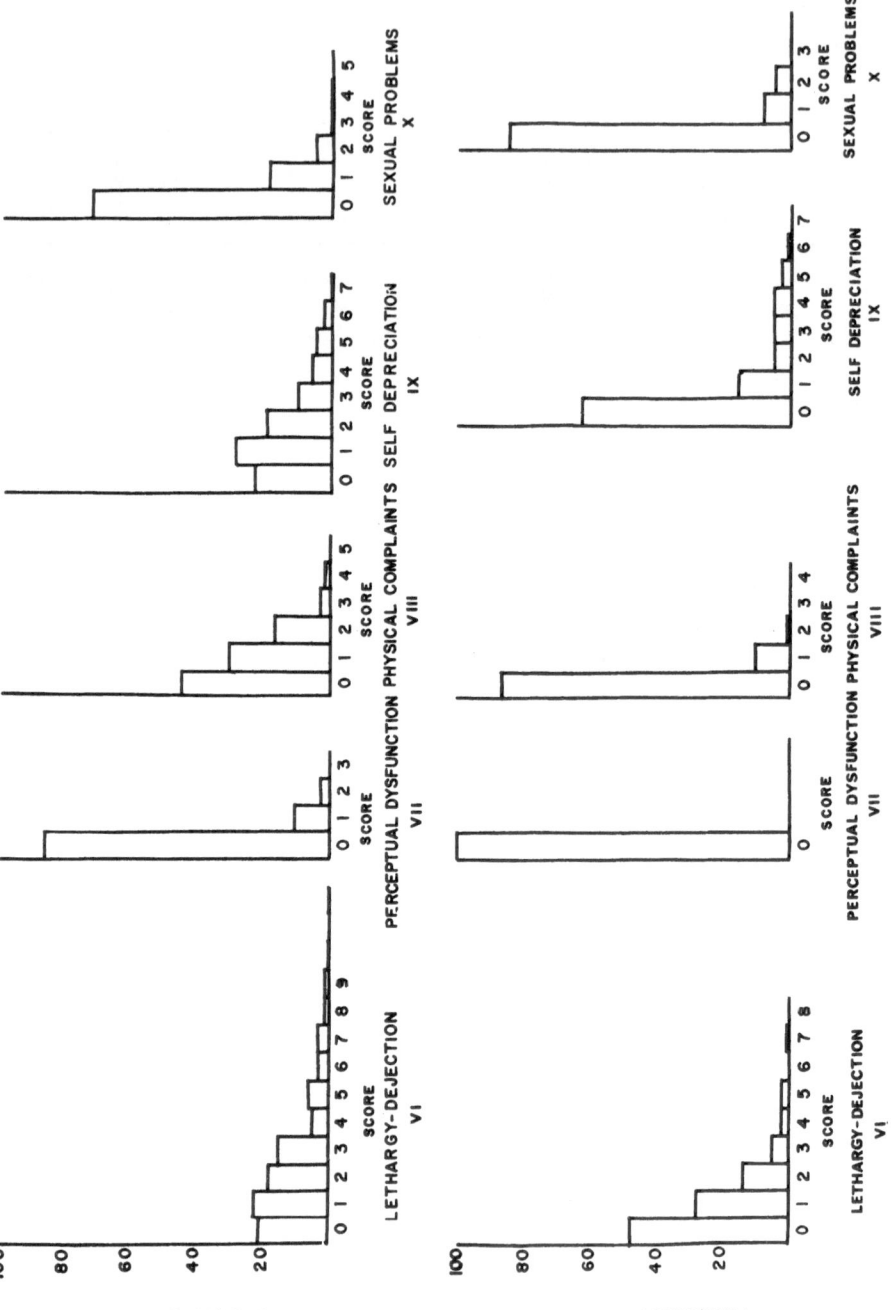

Fig. 8. Frequency distributions of SCI subtest scores of (above) 183 hospitalized mental patients and (below) 95 subjects in the community

18

The individual subtests also show skewed frequency distributions, as can be seen from Figures 7 and 8 in which frequency distributions for each of the ten subtests are presented both for the normals and· the psychiatric patients.

In order to reduce skewness, improve additivity and stabilize the variance, it was considered desirable to transform the raw scores to a new scale. Because the variances of the sample distributions were larger than the means, the negative binomial appeared to be the most appropriate model for the underlying distribution in the population of which the items represent a sample. This is a family of discrete exponential decay functions of the general form $\binom{-k}{n}$ $p^k$ $(-q)^n$ in which the variances are larger than the means. When $k = 1$, the negative binomial reduces to $pq^n$, which is known as the geometric distribution. As a first approximation, the geometric distribution, the simplest of the negative binomial family, was fitted to the total and subtest distributions of the sample of normals. Goodness of fit was tested by chi square on the sample of 48 community subjects.

Table 6. Chi Square Goodness of Fit Tests for the Geometric Distribution of Sample Data from 48 Normals

| Subtest | $\tilde{p}$(=Prob. of score of 0) | $\tilde{q}$(=Prob. of score of 1 or more) | $\chi^2$ | df | p |
|---------|------|------|------|------|------|
| 1 | .9056 | .0944 | .20 | 1 | >.05 |
| 2 | .6667 | .3333 | 1.32 | 1 | >.05 |
| 3 | .8421 | .1579 | 1.50 | 1 | >.05 |
| 4 | .7868 | .2132 | .16 | 1 | >.05 |
| 5 | .9795 | .0205 | 0 | 0 | >.05 |
| 6 | .6400 | .3600 | 2.26 | 2 | >.05 |
| 7 | 1.000 | 0 | 0 | 0 | >.05 |
| 8 | .9056 | .0944 | .06 | 0 | >.05 |
| 9 | .6315 | .3685 | 7.06 | 3 | >.05 |
| 10 | .8275 | .1725 | .69 | 1 | >.05 |
| Total | .2667 | .7333 | 1.37 | 10 | >.05 |

$$\tilde{p} = \frac{N}{N + \sum_{i=0}^{\infty} in_i} , \text{where} \quad N = \text{Total sample size}$$

and $n_i$ = Number of Ss with score of i ($\sum_{i=0}^{\infty} n_i = N$)

19

The results are shown in Table 6. No significant deviations from expectation were noted. A transformation, $\log_e (\sqrt{x} + \sqrt{x+1})$, was derived by Bartlett's (1947) method. As Table 7 reveals, there is a marked decrease in the ratios of variances to means as a result of the transformation.

Table 7. Comparison of Raw and Transformed Scores of a Sample of 95 Normal Subjects

| Subareas | Raw Scores | | Transformed Scores | |
|---|---|---|---|---|
| | $\bar{X}$ | $s^2$ | $\bar{Y}$ [a] | $s^2$ |
| 1. Anger-Hostility | .3789 | .5357 | .2596 | .1976 |
| 2. Conceptual Dysfunction | .3368 | .6726 | .2064 | .1800 |
| 3. Fear-Worry | .3053 | .4058 | .2161 | .1708 |
| 4. Incongruous Behavior | .2211 | .2591 | .1744 | .1339 |
| 5. Incongruous Ideation | .1579 | .1982 | .1197 | .1018 |
| 6. Lethargy-Dejection | .8947 | 1.4143 | .5370 | .2947 |
| 7. Perceptual Dysfunction | 0 | 0 | 0 | 0 |
| 8. Physical Complaints | .1368 | .1406 | .1141 | .0917 |
| 9. Self Depreciation | .8632 | 2.1406 | .4200 | .3313 |
| 10. Sexual Problems | .2000 | .2681 | .1438 | .1234 |
| Total | 3.4947 | 14.8697 | 1.0447 | .4513 |

[a] $Y = \log_e (\sqrt{X} + \sqrt{X+1})$

## STANDARDIZATION

Because the ten subtests contain different numbers of items, the transformed scores of the normals were converted to standard form with mean of zero so as to facilitate profiling of a subject's scores on the different subtests and to allow for comparisons among individuals and groups. Initially, total raw score was transformed and standardized independently of the subtests. However, experience has shown that a more useful procedure is to compute a total score as the mean of the standard scores of the subtests. The total score thus becomes an index of level, i.e., average elevation of the subtests above the norm.

Figure 9 illustrates the method by which the standard scores of clinical groups may be displayed graphically as deviations from the base line of the reference population of normals. The mean of the ten standard scores of the subtests is represented by a bar at the left side of the figure which

20

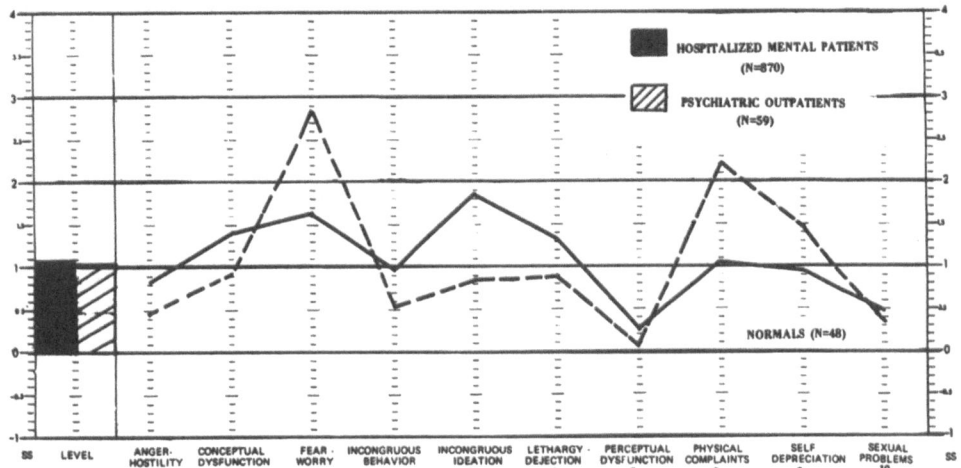

Fig. 9. Comparison of mean scores of inpatients and outpatients

reflects general level of psychopathology. The individual subtests are arranged in alphabetical order and the points representing their standard scores are connected for ease of visualization. For each subtest the mean score of the normals represents the zero point of pathology. Since about 80% of normals obtain scores below one standard deviation, scores higher than one can be regarded as significantly deviant from the norm. Scores lower than zero have no clinical meaning but merely indicate absence of observed pathology in that rubric. The two profiles in Figure 9 show the mean standard scores of two groups of mental patients obtained with an early form of the SCI. The 870 hospitalized mental patients are a mixed sample including chronic residents, first admissions and readmissions. The 59 psychiatric outpatients were interviewed when they visited the psychiatric clinic of a large voluntary hospital. Both groups show significantly elevated levels in the bars at the left of the figure, just above one standard deviation from the norm. Although mean elevation of the two profiles is about the same, there are notable differences in shape. The inpatients show significant elevations (in order of magnitude) in Incongruous Behavior (Subtest 5), Fear-Worry (Subtest 3), Conceptual Dysfunction (Subtest 2), Lethargy-Dejection (Subtest 6), and Physical Complaints (Subtest 8). The outpatients have their peak scores on Fear-Worry (Subtest 3), Physical Complaints (Subtest 8), and Self-Depreciation (Subtest 9).

Figure 10 is similar to Figure 9 in that it shows the mean profiles of a group of inpatients and a group of outpatients based on a zero line made up of the reference population of 95 community subjects. These data, however, were obtained with the current form of the SCI. There are certain differences in the make-up of the normals and of the inpatients which account for the more flattened profiles. The normal group, while twice as large as the

21

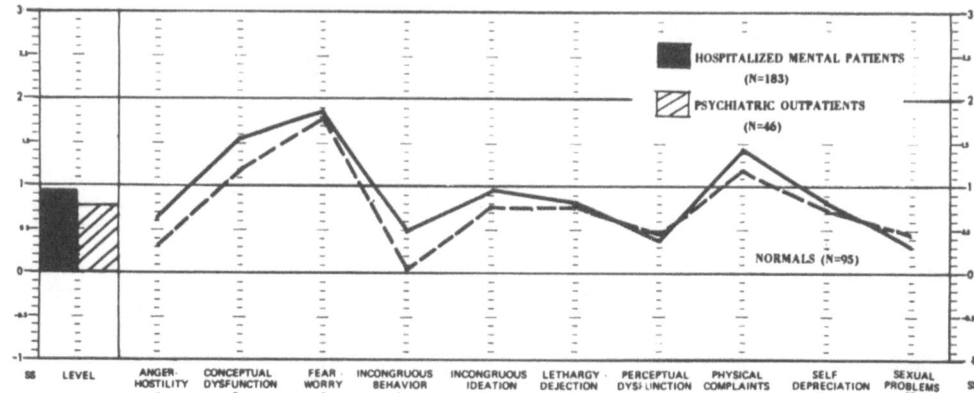

**Fig. 10. Comparison of mean scores of inpatients and outpatients**

earlier sample, is composed entirely of subjects interviewed at a vocational advisement agency. Persons who come for vocational guidance often suffer from psychological impairment, as was indeed verified in several of these cases. Thus the flattened profiles of the two groups of psychiatric patients probably represent an elevation of the zero line, i.e., the new norms are more conservative in assessment of psychopathology than the earlier norms. Moreover, the inpatients are now all recent admissions to a small, therapy-oriented psychiatric hospital. That they are much more similar to outpatients can be seen from the similar shapes of the two profiles. Both inpatients and outpatients peak significantly on Fear-Worry (Subtest 3), Conceptual Dysfunction (Subtest 2), and Physical Complaints (Subtest 8).

OTHER REFERENCE GROUPS

In order to determine the suitability of the SCI for younger subjects, a sample of persons 16 and 17 years of age was drawn from a vocational advisement agency. Thirty-two of these were males, 17 females. In Table 8 their mean raw scores are presented along with those of the two earlier samples of adult normals. On the average, the adolescent group shows lower scores, so that separate norms are necessary for subjects in the younger age groups. Such norms have been constructed from the above sample of adolescents by applying the transformation and standardization procedure used for the adult samples.

Two samples of physically ill subjects have been examined with the SCI for the purpose of assessing the sensitivity of the technique for the psychological disturbances attributable to physical illness. The first of these was a group of ten patients suspected of having cancer who were interviewed on their first visit to a cancer clinic. Their mean scores are shown in Figure 11. Although the mean level of pathology is within the normal range, as shown by the bar at the left of the figure, they show significantly elevated scores on Fear-Worry (Subtest 3) and on Physical Complaints

22

Table 8. Raw Scores and Standard Deviations for Three Groups of Community Subjects on the SCI

| SUBTEST | (N=48) [1] | | (N=95) | | (N=49) [2] | |
|---|---|---|---|---|---|---|
| | X̄ | s | X̄ | s | X̄ | s |
| | 2.91 | 3.40 | 3.49 | 3.86 | 2.00 | 2.47 |
| 1 | .31 | .72 | .37 | .73 | .33 | .85 |
| 2 | .52 | .71 | .34 | .82 | .31 | .80 |
| 3 | .19 | .57 | .31 | .64 | .18 | .53 |
| 4 | .33 | .60 | .22 | .51 | .08 | .34 |
| 5 | .13 | .39 | .16 | .45 | 0 | 0 |
| 6 | .56 | .87 | .89 | 1.19 | .63 | 1.05 |
| 7 | 0 | 0 | 0 | 0 | 0 | 0 |
| 8 | .10 | .37 | .14 | .38 | .06 | .24 |
| 9 | .58 | 1.18 | .86 | 1.46 | .33 | .99 |
| 10 | .19 | .57 | .20 | .52 | .08 | .28 |

[1] Preliminary form

[2] 17 - 18 year olds

(Subtest 8). In Figure 12 is shown the profile of a group of patients who were suffering from intractable pain. They were interviewed the day before they were to submit to a percutaneous chordotomy, a surgical procedure for relief of pain. Mean level of psychopathology is within the normal limits, but there are significantly elevated scores on Physical Complaints (Subtest 8), almost three standard deviations above the mean; Incongruous Behavior (Subtest 4), which includes unusual or bizarre gestures and mannerisms; Fear-Worry (Subtest 3); and Self-Depreciation (Subtest 8), which includes feelings of worthlessness, regret, and inferiority.

## STABILITY

Determination of stability by the test-retest method presents special problems for a technique like the SCI, which is sensitive to short-term fluctuations in behavioral adaptation. It might be expected, however, that continuously hospitalized chronic psychotics would show relatively little change in

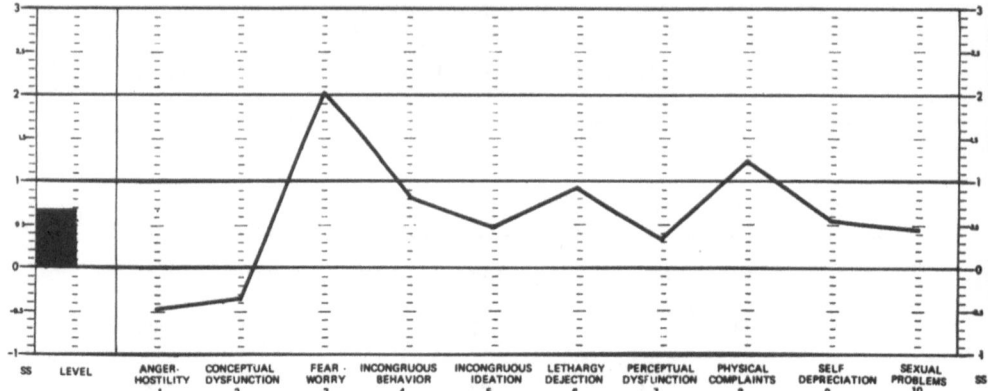

Fig. 11. Mean scores of 10 patients suspected of having cancer who were interviewed on first visit to a cancer clinic

adaptation over time. A small sample of nine chronic resident patients from a study of chronic schizophrenics (Burdock & Hardesty, 1966) was reinterviewed after six months. These patients had been transferred from the regular continued treatment services of a large state mental hospital to a special intensive treatment unit and had been returned to the regular services because of failure to show sufficient improvement to warrant release. A product-moment correlation of .84 was obtained between total scores for the two occasions. Fisher's z-transformation provided 95% confidence limits as follows: $.40 < r > .97$. Figure 13 shows the mean profiles of the subtest scores for the first and follow-up interviews. The lower initial scores of these patients may have been caused by the extra attention they received at the time of their transfer into the intensive treatment unit.

### Interviewer Effects

The effect of different interviewers on the responses of the subject was examined on a sample of 22 newly admitted, carefully diagnosed schizophrenics. Diagnosis had been made independently by the psychiatrist. Eleven of the patients were interviewed by a male interviewer, the other 11 by a female interviewer. Mean profiles of the two groups of patients are compared

Fig. 12. Mean scores of 7 patients with intractable pain who were interviewed the day before receiving percutaneous chordotomy

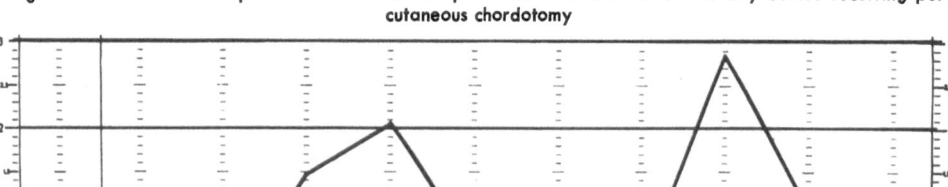

24

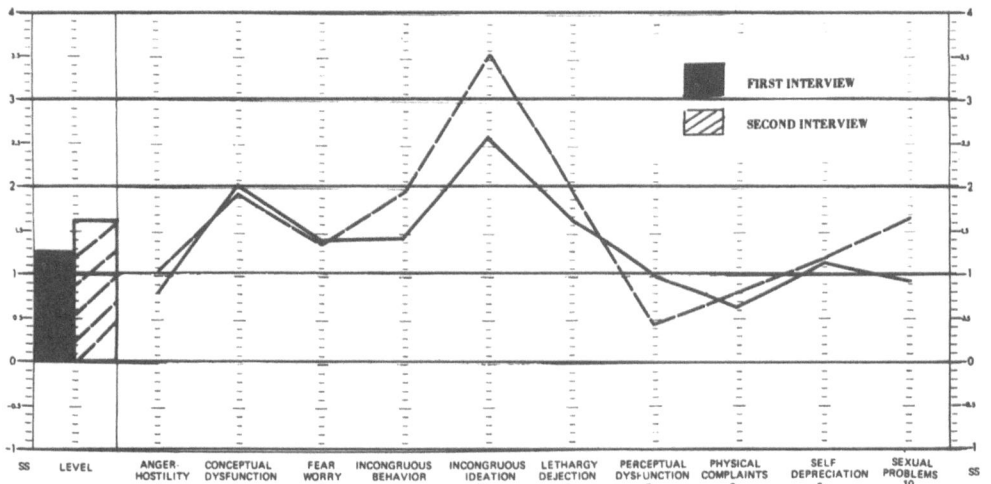

Fig. 13. Test-retest profiles of a group of nine continuously hospitalized chronic schizophrenics reinterviewed after six months

in Figure 14. Differences in level and profile are comparatively minor.

CONCURRENT VALIDITY

Initial evidence for the validity of the SCI total score was obtained from correlations of SCI total scores with the *Ward Behavior Inventory* (Burdock & Hardesty, 1968). A correlation of .68 was found on a sample of 16 resident mental patients. Fisher's r to z transformation yielded 95% confidence limits for the population r of .28 to .88. On a sample of newly admitted mental patients a correlation of .35 was obtained between the SCI total score and the WBI. The 95% confidence limits gave a population r between .13 and .54.

Fig. 14. Acute schizophrenics interviewed by a male and a female interviewer respectively

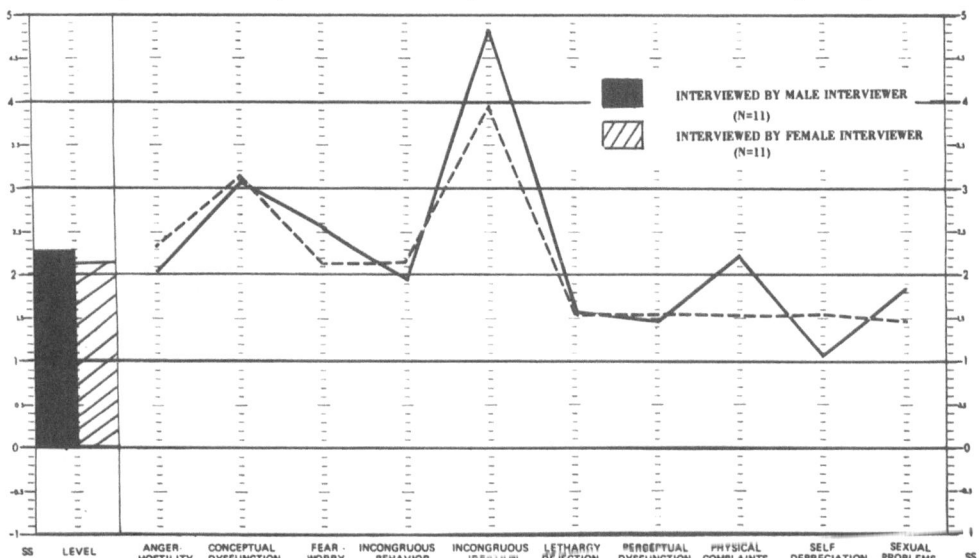

25

In a study with a preliminary form of the SCI, 52 schizophrenics from the back wards of a state mental hospital were interviewed at the time that they were transferred into an intensive treatment unit. By the end of a month, 12 of the patients had been returned to the back wards because they failed to respond to treatment. The mean of the total scores for these 12 patients was significantly higher, i.e., indicative of more pathology, than the mean score of the 40 patients retained under treatment. The relevant data may be seen in Table 9.

Table 9. Comparison of SCI Total Scores of Improved and Unimproved Chronic Schizophrenics (1961)

| Group | Mean | Standard Deviation |
|---|---|---|
| Improved   (N=40) | 15.2 | 5.7 |
| Unimproved   (N=12) | 24.1 | 9.9 |

$t = 8.83$,   $p < .001$

## Differences among Clinical Groups

Figure 15a presents a comparison of the mean standard scores of a sample of 12 manic patients with a sample of 18 depressed patients, all of whom were interviewed on admission to a psychiatric receiving hospital. The total scores, shown by the bars at the left of the profile, indicate that both groups exceed the nonpsychiatric reference group in overall morbidity, and that they are closely similar in this respect. However, the two profiles have certain characteristic differences which distinguish the two diagnostic groups. The solid line profile of the depressives contrasts sharply with the broken-line profile of the manics. The following features may be noted. The depressives display no Anger-Hostility (Subtest 1), while the manics in contrast show a significant elevation in this area. Both groups display significant amounts of Conceptual Dysfunction (Subtest 2), but the manics have about twice as much as the depressives. Fear-Worry (Subtest 3) is significant for both groups but much higher among the depressives. Incongruous Behavior (Subtest 4) shows an appreciable elevation for both manics and depressives. The manics show a very high elevation on Incongruous Ideation (Subtest 5), but the depressives are within the normal range. Lethargy-Dejection (Subtest 6) separates the two groups, as might have been anticipated intuitively. Thus the depressives show a high elevation in this area, while the manics are

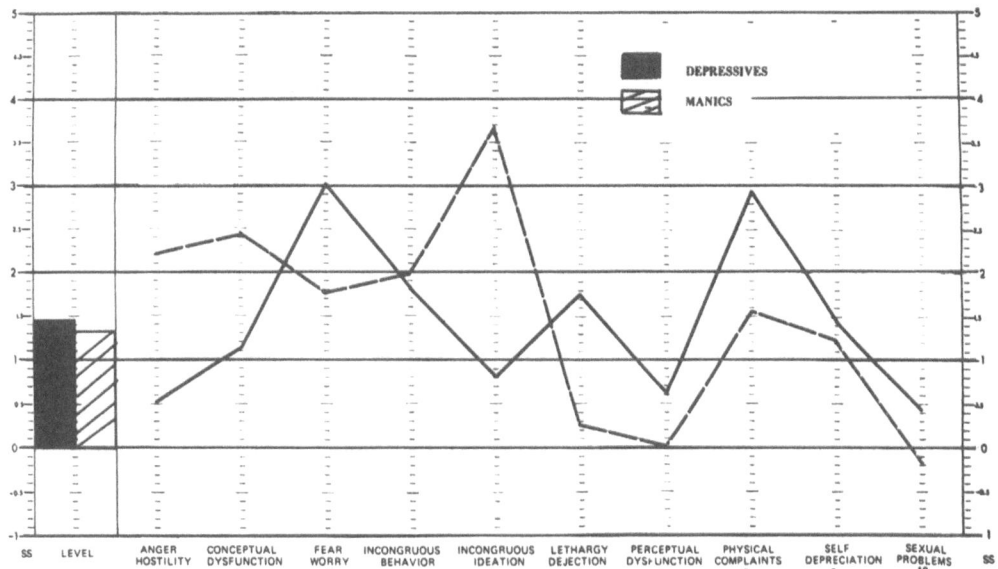

Fig. 15a. Comparison of mean standard scores of a sample of 12 manic patients with a sample of 18 depressed patients interviewed on admission to a psychiatric receiving hospital

within the normal range. In the area of Perceptual Dysfunction (Subtest 7), neither group shows a significant elevation. In Physical Complaints (Subtest 8), both groups show a significant elevation, but the depressives make much higher scores. On Self Depreciation (Subtest 9) both groups show elevations above the normal. Neither group shows a significant score on Sexual Problems (Subtest 10). In summary, the manics are distinguished from the depressives by significantly higher elevations in Anger-Hostility, Conceptual Dysfunction, and Incongruous Ideation, and by significantly less Fear-Worry and Lethargy-Dejection where the depressives correspondingly show the higher elevations.

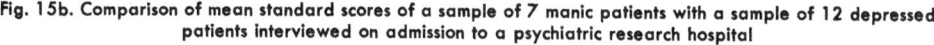

Fig. 15b. Comparison of mean standard scores of a sample of 7 manic patients with a sample of 12 depressed patients interviewed on admission to a psychiatric research hospital

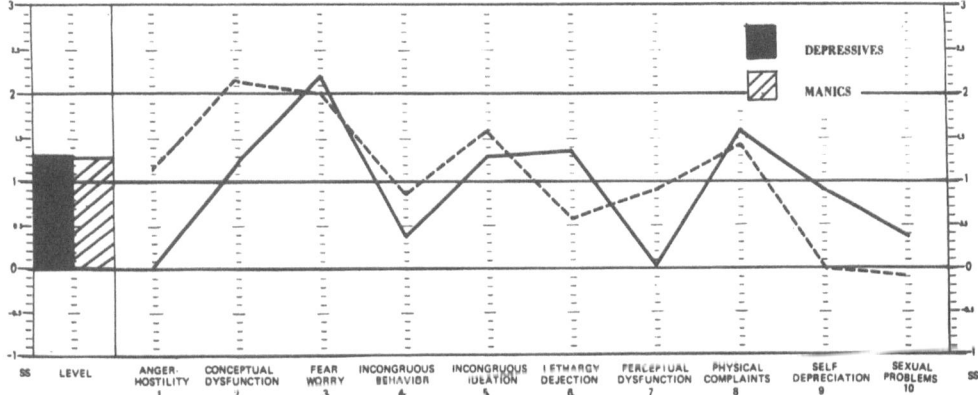

*Institutional differences.* As an example of how institutional differences are reflected on the SCI, Figure 15b displays profiles of seven manics and 12 depressives from a psychiatric research hospital. Although the two diagnostic groups show about the same characteristic differences in pattern, the profiles are closer together and much less elevated at the research hospital than at the receiving hospital, which is a catchall for the most difficult patients.

Figure 16 illustrates contrasting profiles of small homogeneous groups who were interviewed on admission to a research ward. Diagnosis was made independently of the interview. The solid bar and line show the mean level and profile of a group of clearcut, carefully diagnosed, inpatient schizophrenics. Their mean level is more than two deviation units above that of normals and the whole profile is elevated above the range of random variation. The highest scores for this group are in Incongruous Ideation (Subtest 5), Conceptual Dysfunction (Subtest 2), Incongruous Behavior (Subtest 4), Fear-Worry (Subtest 3), and Anger-Hostility (Subtest 1). Moreover, the significant elevation on Perceptual Dysfunction (Subtest 7), is almost pathognomonic for schizophrenia. The dashed bar and profile are for the depressives, a group independently diagnosed for the research ward with the same careful procedure as that used for the schizophrenics. They show a lower mean level of pathology than the schizophrenics in the bar at the left of the figure, but nevertheless, a significantly elevated level. The peak points in their profile are Fear-Worry (Subtest 3), Physical Complaints (Subtest 8), Lethargy-Dejection (Subtest 6), and Self Depreciation (Subtest 9). Unlike the schizophrenics, the depressives are within the normal range for Anger-Hostility (Subtest 1), Incongruous Ideation (Subtest 5), Perceptual Dysfunction (Subtest 7) and Sexual Problems (Subtest 10). They show a com-

Fig. 16. Comparison of mean SCI scores of depressives and schizophrenics

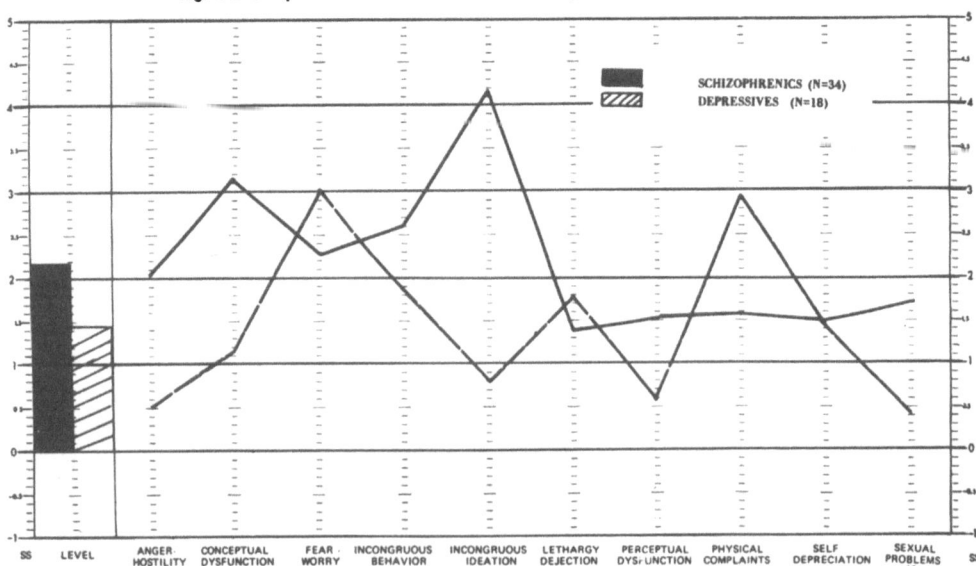

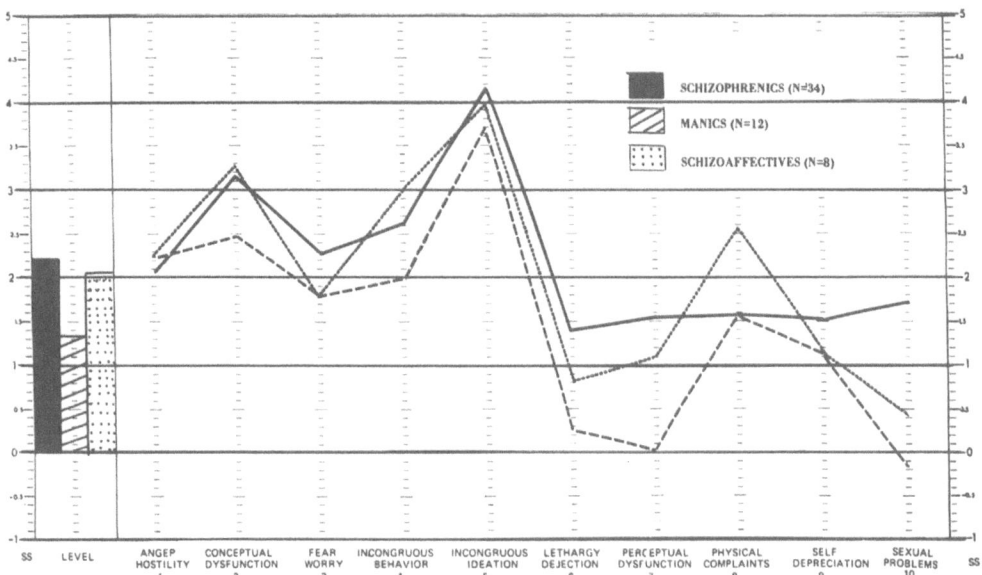

Fig. 17. Comparison of mean scores of schizoaffectives with those of manics and schizophrenics

parable amount of Self Depreciation (Subtest 9) and significant but lesser amounts of Incongruous Behavior (Subtest 4) and Conceptual Dysfunction (Subtest 2).

A recurrent problem in psychiatric diagnosis is that of distinguishing schizoaffectives from manics (Burdock & Hardesty, 1969). In Figure 17 the solid line (and bar) of the schizophrenic sample is again reproduced, but now it is contrasted with a dashed line profile of a sample of 12 manics and an X-ed line profile of a group of eight schizoaffectives. Corresponding bar graphs for level of pathology appear on the left side of the figure and show the manics, as a group, to be at a slightly lower level of pathology than the other two groups. All SCI assessments reflect admission status and were made independently of diagnosis, the separation into diagnostic groupings being made subsequently. In contrast to the schizoaffectives, whose profile follows that of the other schizophrenics fairly closely, the manics show no evidence of Sexual Problems (Subtest 10), Lethargy-Dejection (Subtest 6) or Perceptual Dysfunction (Subtest 7). A high score on this rubic, as pointed out earlier, is almost pathognomonic for schizophrenia, and thus for schizoaffectives.

Figure 18 displays the mean profile of a group of five outpatients who had chronic brain syndrome. There is a significant elevation in level of pathology as shown by the bar at the left. Among the subtests the highest elevations are on Physical Complaints (Subtest 8) and Conceptual Dysfunction (Subtest 2), both of which are more than two and one-half standard deviations from the norm. Lesser but significant elevations are also shown on Fear-Worry (Subtest 3), Self Depreciation (Subtest 9) and Lethargy-Dejection (Subtest 6).

29

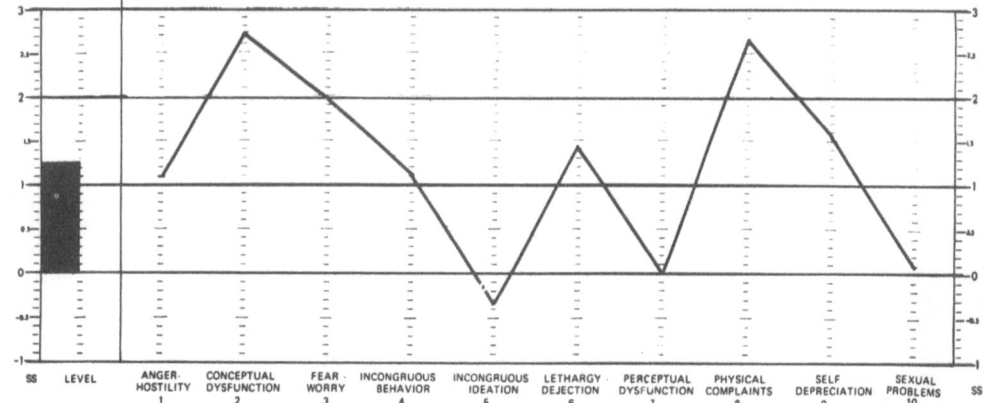

Fig. 18. Mean SCI profile of a group of 5 outpatients with chronic brain syndrome

There is also some evidence of Incongruous Behavior (Subtest 4) and Anger-Hostility (Subtest 1).

### PROFILE CHANGES AFTER TREATMENT

In Figure 19 the same schizophrenics are shown whose mean scores were compared with those of a group of depressives in Figure 16 and with groups of manics and of schizoaffectives in Figure 17. Now they are divided among the three treatment groups to which they were randomly assigned at admission. As these profiles make clear, pretreatment differences among the three groups are not marked either in level of pathology (bar graphs on the left of the figure) or in the configuration of the subtests, although the placebo group tends to be somewhat higher than the others.

In Figure 20 the solid bar and line once again depict the pretreatment level

Fig. 19. Pretreatment profiles of newly admitted acute schizophrenics subsequently assigned to three different drugs

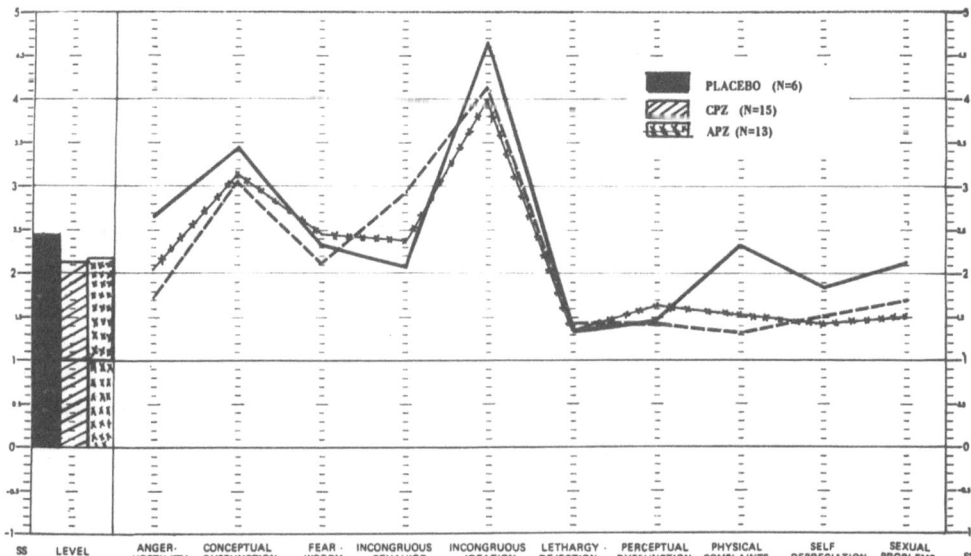

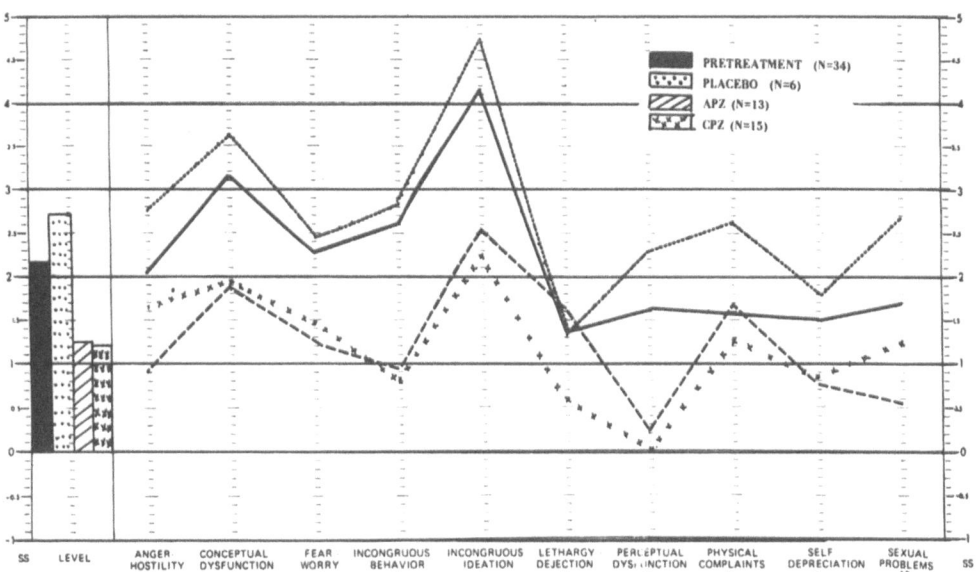

Fig. 20. Follow-up profiles of acute schizophrenics after one month on three different treatments

and profile of the combined groups. The other three profiles show the relative statuses of the three treatment groups after one month. The placebo group (dotted bar and line) shows no improvement; on the contrary, severity of symptoms has increased in almost all areas. The other two treatment groups, acetophenazine (dashed bar and line) and chlorpromazine (X's), both show approximately equal declines in level of pathology to nearly normal. In both groups, Incongruous Behavior (Subtest 4), Perceptual Dysfunction (Subtest 7) and Self Depreciation (Subtest 9) have come within the normal range. The acetophenazine group drops to within the normal range in Anger-Hostility (Subtest 1) and in Sexual Problems (Subtest 10), while the chlorpromazine group shows a less significant decline on these two subtests. On the other hand, the chlorpromazine group shows a unique drop in Lethargy-Dejection (Subtest 6), whereas the acetophenazine group shows no improvement at all on this rubric. This finding runs counter to the usual expectation that piperazine phenothiazines are more effective than chlorpromazine in reducing apathy and retardation. A report by Goldberg and Mattsson (1968) provides some independent corroboration for this result. They found that "apathy and retardation predicts improvement . . . in chlorpromazine treated patients [contrary to] the general folklore on drug specificity. . . ."

Figures 21 and 22 show the Before-and-After profiles of the schizoaffectives who were divided into two groups treated with chlorpromazine and lithium respectively. The group treated with chlorpromazine shows, after two weeks, a slight diminution in level, a drop in Conceptual Dysfunction (Subtest 2), which, however, remains elevated above the normal range, and a decline in Lethargy-Dejection (Subtest 6) to within the normal range, as was found in the case of schizophrenics treated with CPZ. Surprisingly, the schizoaffectives

31

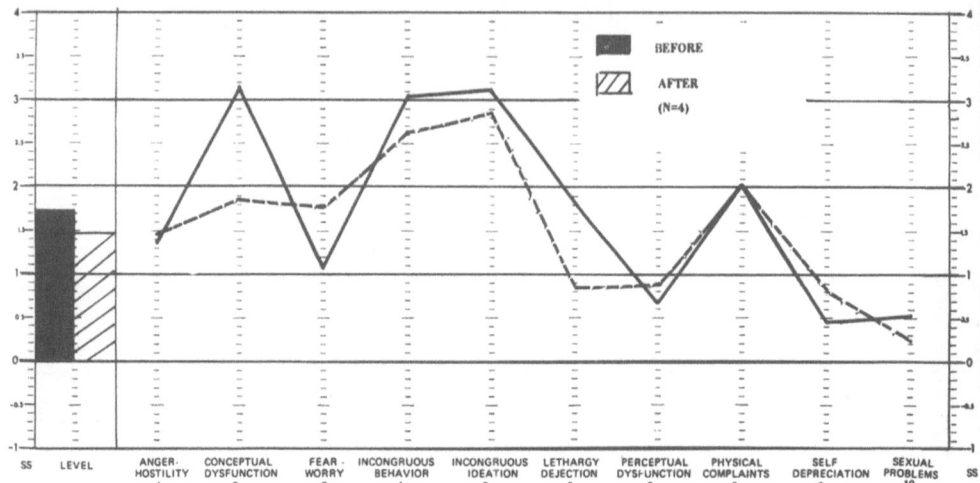

Fig. 21. Profiles of schizoaffectives treated with cpz

treated with lithium, though sicker or admission (two and one-half deviation units above normal level as compared with one and three-quarters units for the CPZ group) show a more marked drop, almost to normal level. Perhaps they had more room to travel. Fear-Worry (Subtest 3), Self Depreciation (Subtest 9) and Sexual Problems (Subtest 10) appear to be dissipated, and Anger-Hostility (Subtest 1) and Conceptual Dysfunction (Subtest 2) drop nearly to the normal range. Significantly, Perceptual Dysfunction (Subtest 7) remains high, apparently impervious to treatment. Despite similar diagnoses, the two treatment groups show certain pretreatment differences which might account for differences in response to treatment: the CPZ group starts with a significant amount of Lethargy-Dejection (Subtest 6) whose

Fig. 22. Profiles of schizoaffectives treated with lithium

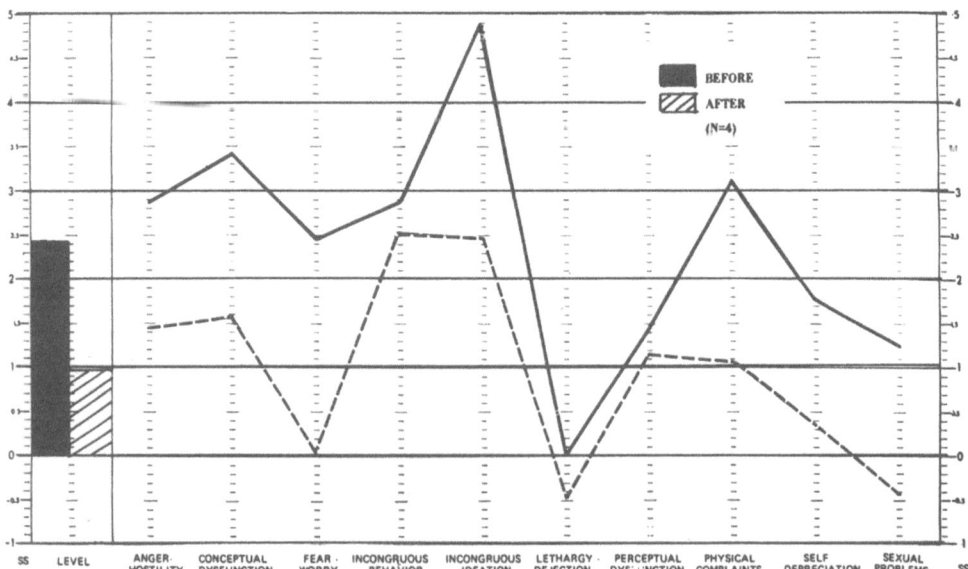

32

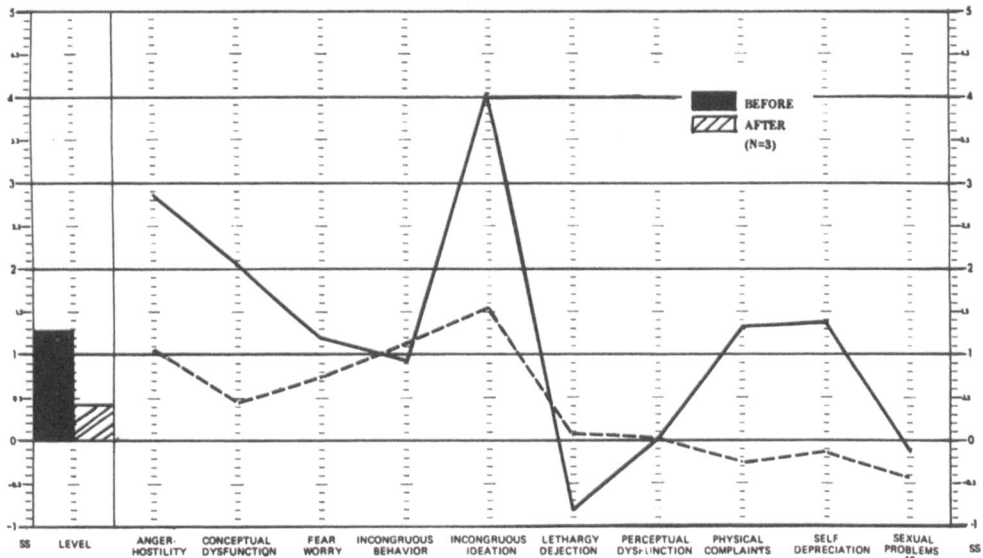

Fig. 23. Follow-up profiles of manics treated with cpz for two weeks

reduction by treatment is accompanied by a rise in Fear-Worry (Subtest 3), while the lithium group starts and ends with no evidence of Lethargy-Dejection (Subtest 6), but retains its initial Perceptual Dysfunction (Subtest 7).

In Figures 23 and 24, the manics previously shown in Figure 19 are divided into the same two treatment groups as the schizoaffectives. The two manic groups start at about the same level of pathology. Both treatments are accompanied by a decline to the normal range, although the CPZ group shows a somewhat greater drop.

With respect to schizophrenia, the data presented here indicate that individuals classified as schizophrenics can be characterized in explicit and quantifiable terms by those behavioral elements which are critical for the diagnosis.

Fig. 24. Follow-up profiles of manics treated with lithuim for two weeks

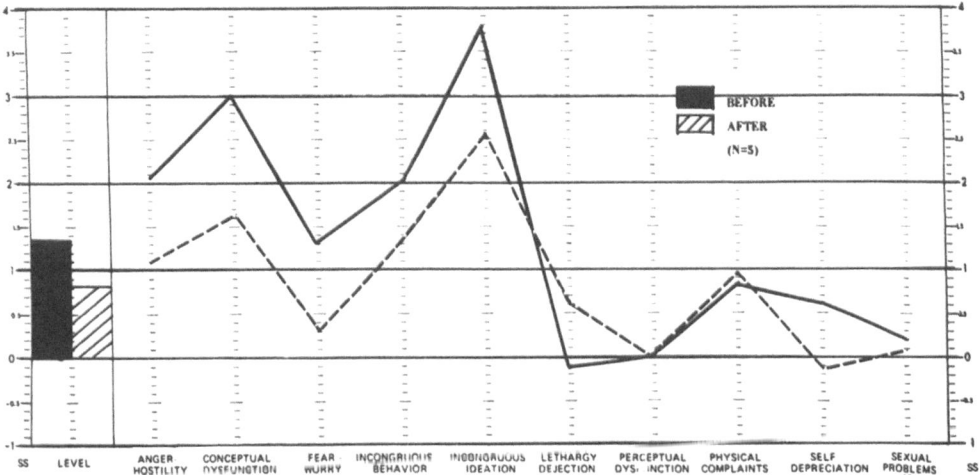

33

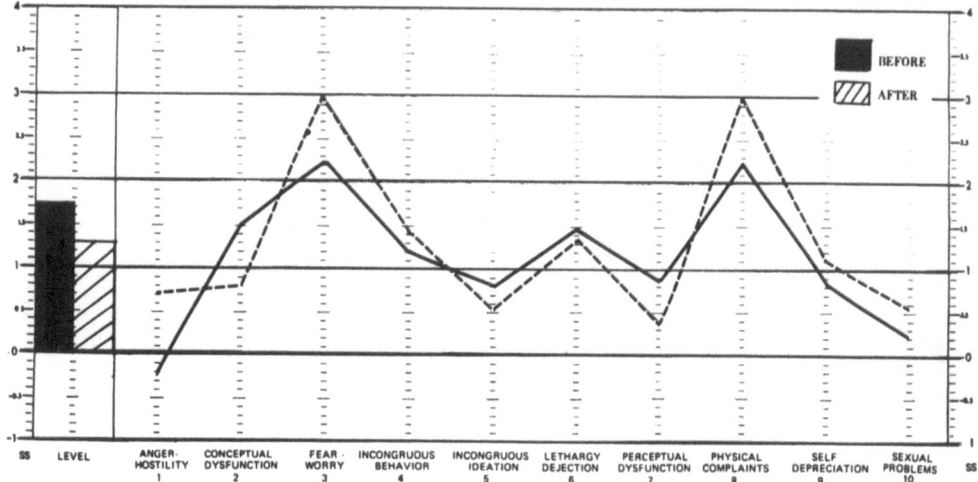

Fig. 25. Before-and-after treatment profiles of 10 depressives treated with an experimental drug

The data also indicate that improvement in schizophrenics treated by phenothiazines tends to be represented by a general downward drift in psychopathology, i.e., a decline in level of pathology rather than a change in the specific characteristics of the illness. In manic-depressive psychosis, on the other hand, the behaviors at opposite ends of the cycle seem like mirror images of one another (see Figures 15a and 15b).

Figure 25 displays the before (solid line) and after (broken line) mean profiles of a sample of ten patients who were treated with an experimental drug. Severity of illness before treatment is deflected in a total score more than one-and-a-half standard deviations above the norm. There is a small decline in overall severity of symptoms after treatment, but the total score remains significantly elevated. Chief features of the pretreatment profile are significantly elevated scores on five of the ten subtests. These are (in order of magnitude): Fear-Worry and Physical Complaints (almost three standard deviations above the norm), Lethargy-Dejection (ca. two standard deviations above the norm), Incongruous Behavior and Self Depreciation. All of these show small diminutions after treatment but, except for Self Depreciation, they remain significantly elevated above the norm. There is, however, a significant rise in Conceptual Dysfunction, and small increases in Incongruous Ideation and Perceptual Dysfunction.

All of the patients in this study had a psychiatric diagnosis of depression and were treated with an experimental drug to ascertain its efficacy as an antidepressant. It is noteworthy that the pretreatment SCI profile shows its most significant elevations on the subtests for Fear-Worry, Physical Complaints and Lethargy-Dejection and that there are also significant elevations in Incongruous Behavior and Self Depreciation. The first three of these are characteristically observed in the profiles of depressives. The high score on

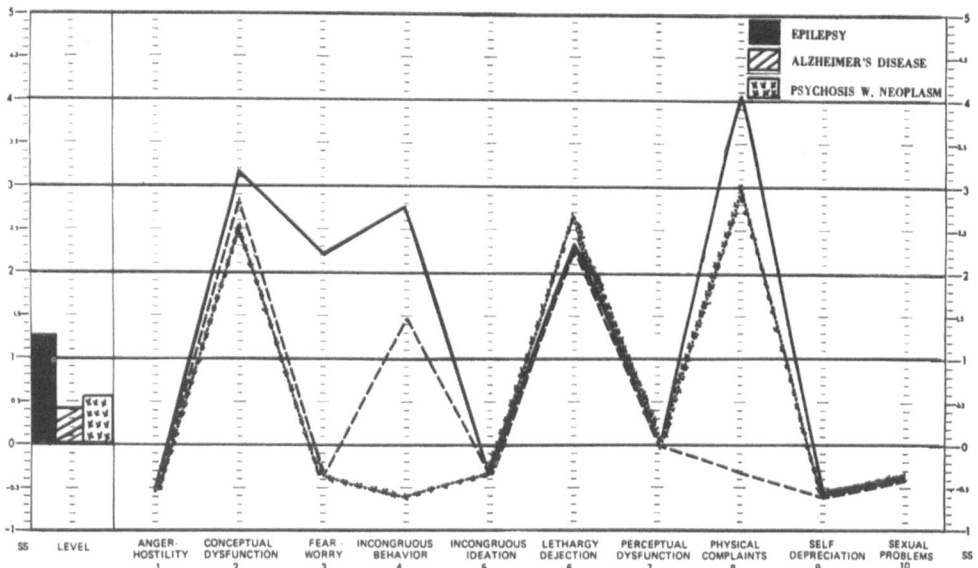

Fig. 26. SCI profiles of three mental patients with organic disease

Incongruous Behavior is, however, a peculiarity of this sample rather than of depressives in general.

In view of the relatively small change in the depressive features of the profile after treatment, which is offset by the significant rise in Conceptual Dysfunction and the increases in Incongruous Ideation and Perceptual Dysfunction, one may reasonably conclude that the experimental drug did not produce a therapeutic change in the group studied. This conclusion is corroborated by the independent clinical judgments of the team of psychiatrists in charge of the study.

INDIVIDUAL CASES

Figure 26 illustrates how the SCI can be used to compare individual subjects. The base line represents the mean scores of the norm group of non-psychiatric subjects. The three organics represented here were interviewed at time of admission to the hospital. The epileptic is the only one of the three with a significantly elevated total score. All three patients show a lack of Anger-Hostility and Incongruous Ideation, but elevated scores on Conceptual Dysfunction and Lethargy-Dejection. These features are consistent with expectancies expressed in the clinical literature. Other common features of the three profiles are low scores on Perceptual Dysfunction and Self Depreciation.

Figure 27 presents successive profiles of a female manic-depressive patient given lithium therapy who was interviewed three times at intervals of two months. The first interview took place on admission to hospital, the second interview two months later at the time of a marked change in the patient's behavior. The third interview was held two months after the second, on a

35

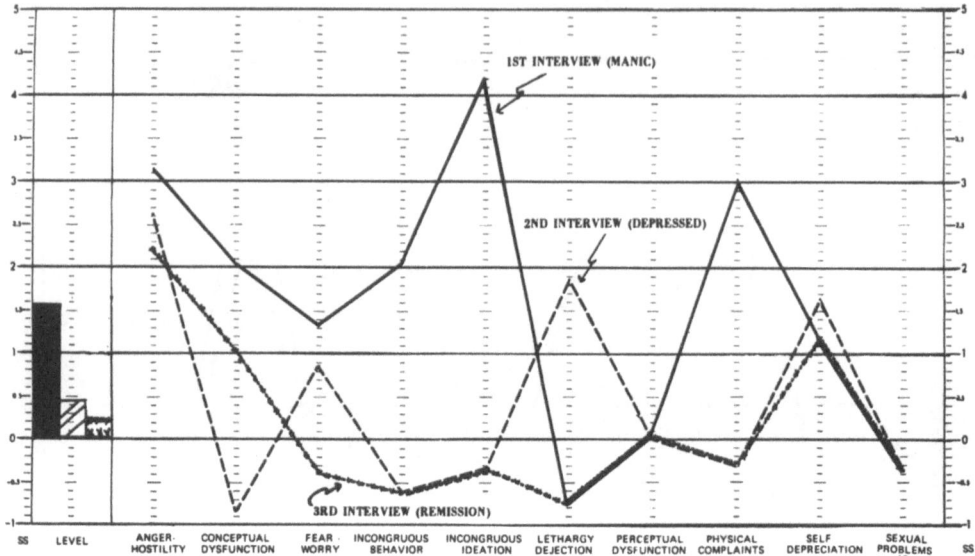

Fig. 27. SCI profiles of a manic-depressive patient treated with lithium who was interviewed three times at bimonthly intervals

follow-up visit by the patient who had been released in the interim. The three total scores show a progressive decline in overall level of psychopathology from a high of one-and-a-half standard deviations above normal to less than one. The profile of subtest scores shows two features which remain relatively high on all three occasions: Anger-Hostility and Self Depreciation. In her manic phase at time of admission, the patient showed extreme Incongruous Ideation and had numerous Physical Complaints. She also manifested considerable Conceptual Dysfunction, Incongruous Behavior, and Fear-Worry. Two months later, in a depressed phase, Incongruous Ideation, Conceptual

Fig. 28. Manic-depressive patient interviewed three times at different phases of illness

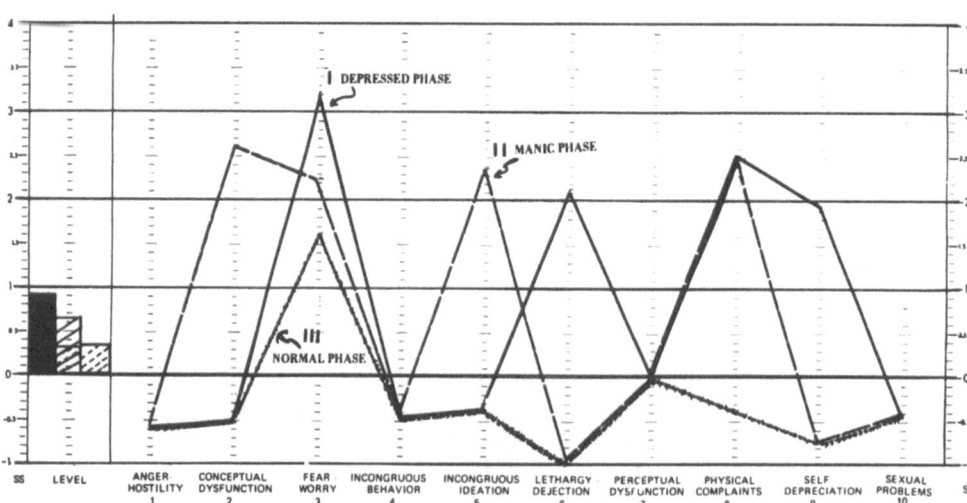

Dysfunction, and Incongruous Behavior, together with Physical Complaints, had all declined to normal, but Lethargy-Dejection had risen. By the time of the follow-up interview, Fear-Worry had returned to normal, but Conceptual Dysfunction had increased again to a significant extent and, together with Anger-Hostility and Self Depreciation, reflects the persistency of deviation from the normal reference group.

Figures 28 and 29 show another manic-depressive patient who was interviewed at each phase of illness during two successive cycles. The first episode ran from mid-June to the end of July; the second episode started early in November and ended in the first part of February. This patient was treated with a combination of Parnate and Elavil for her depression and with lithium for her manic condition. The two sets of profiles give a striking illustration of the similarity of the two cycles.

### PSYCHONEUROTICS

Mean profile for a group of 12 psychoneurotic outpatients is presented in Figure 30. Level of pathology is within the normal range, not surprising for outpatients, but there are significant elevations on Fear-Worry (Subtest 3) and Physical Complaints (Subtest 8). The patients were diagnosed as suffering either from anxiety reaction or reactive depression.

### DRUG ABUSE

A sample of chronic drug users has been interviewed in the community through the intercession of an informant to whom confidentiality had been

**Fig. 29. Same manic-depressive patient during second cycle of illness**

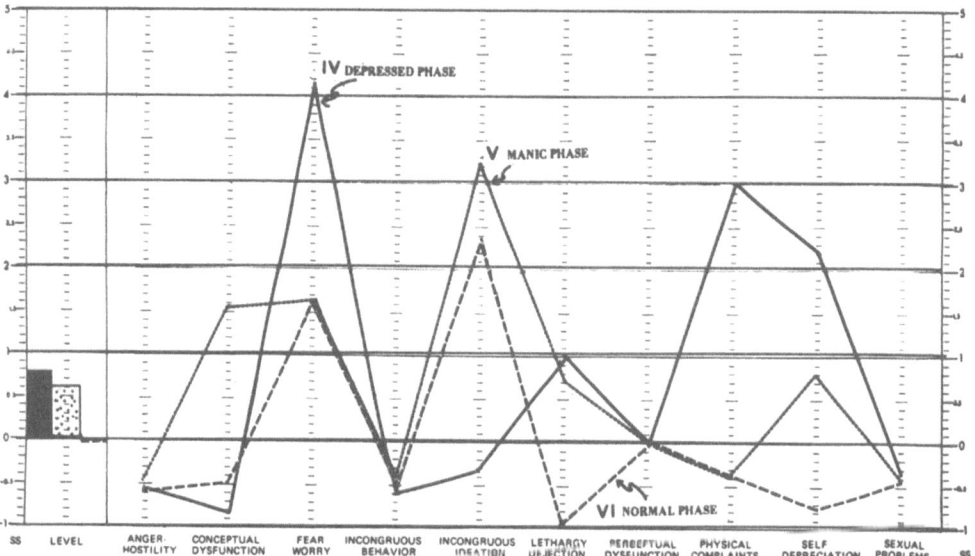

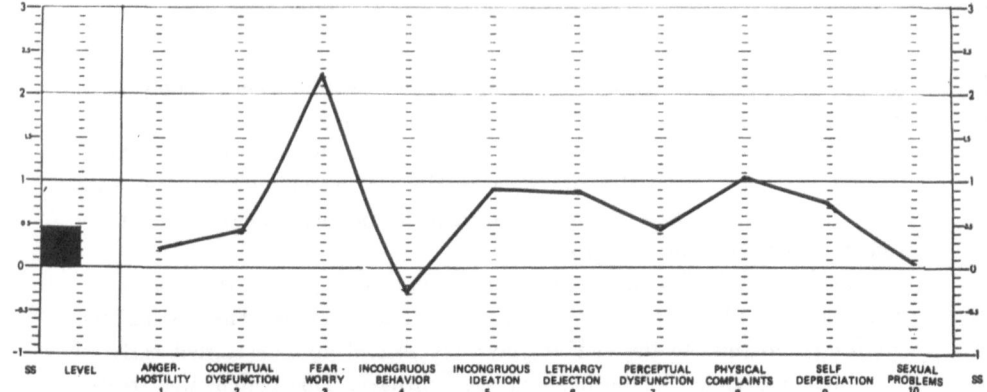

Fig. 30. Mean profile of a group of 12 psychoneurotic outpatients

pledged. Their SCI level is within the normal range, but the mean profile shows some significant elevations above normal expectancy. They are more than two standard deviations from the norm in Incongruous Behavior (Subtest 4) and just over one standard deviation from the norm in Conceptual Dysfunction (Subtest 2), Fear-Worry (Subtest 3), Incongruous Ideation (Subtest 5) and Perceptual Dysfunction (Subtest 7). Their profile, illustrated in Figure 31, is contrasted with that of a small group of patients hospitalized for drug abuse. The latter show a significantly elevated level of pathology, about one-and-a-half standard deviations from the norm. Moreover, their mean profile is somewhat different from that of the community drug users. Thus while they fail to show the Incongruous Behavior (Subtest 4) exhibited by the community group, they are much higher on Incongruous Ideation (Subtest 5) which, it will be recalled, includes delusions and ideas of reference. They also suffer from Lethargy-Dejection (Subtest 6), Physical Complaints (Subtest 8), perhaps due to side effects of the drugs, and Self Depreciation (Subtest 9), i.e., feelings of worthlessness or guilt.

Fig. 31. SCI profiles of two samples of drug users

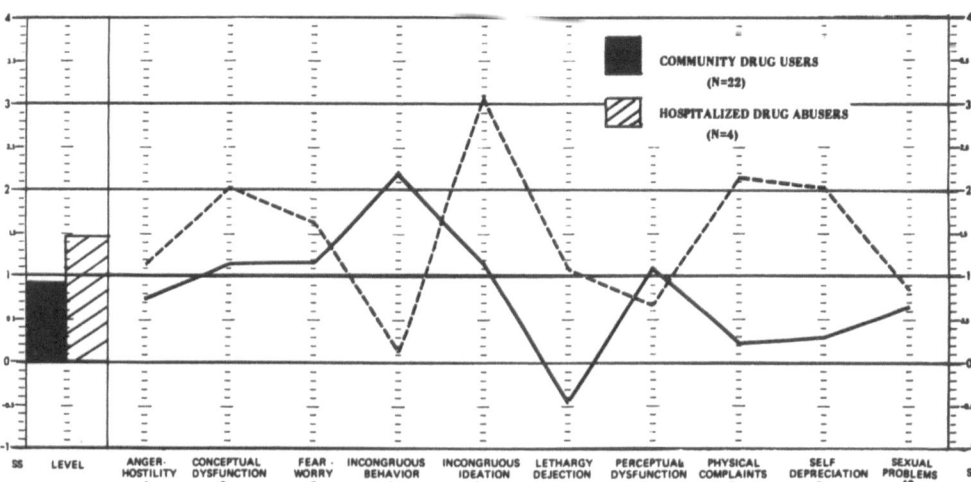

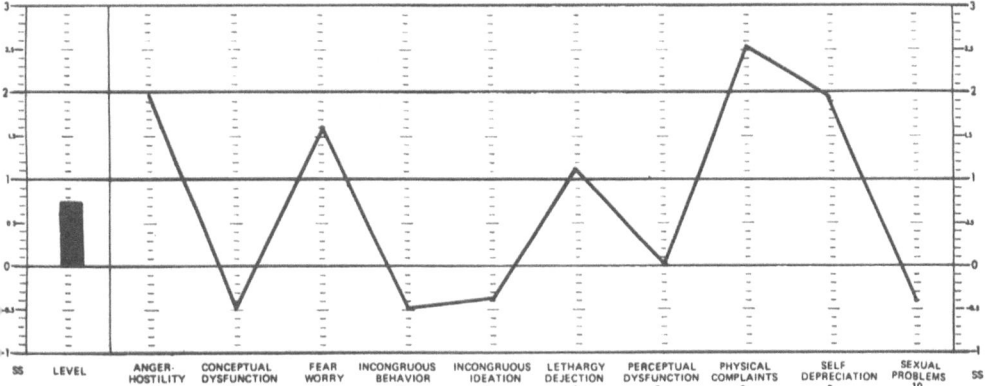

Fig. 32. Profile of a community subject with significantly elevated scores

## SCREENING

Because the interview has been purposely designed to have the quality of an informal inquiry rather than an insistent interrogation, the SCI is peculiarly suited to screening in the general population. Although brief and nondirective in tone, the interview provides a systematic and comprehensive coverage of areas of potential psychopathology. Figures 32 and 33 present profiles of two subjects from the community interviewed in the course of normative studies. Neither subject shows an elevated level of pathology. However, the first subject, a 24-year-old elevator operator, shows significantly elevated scores on Physical Complaints (Subtest 8), Self Depreciation (Subtest 3) and Lethargy-Dejection (Subtest 6). In any screening program such a subject should be referred for more detailed examination. The second subject shows an extremely elevated score on Conceptual Dysfunction (Subtest 2), and almost

Fig. 33. Profile of a community subject subsequently found to have brain damage

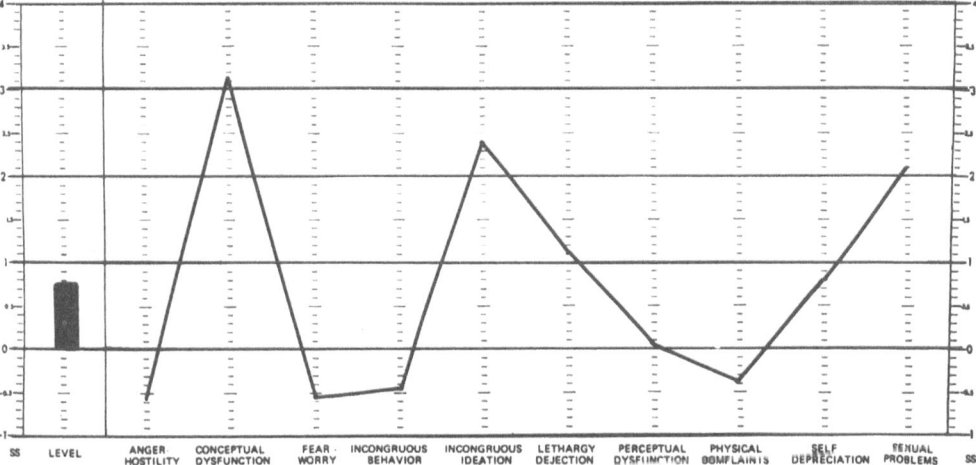

equally high elevations on Incongruous Ideation (Subtest 5) and Sexual Problems (Subtest 10), as well as a significantly high score on Lethargy-Dejection (Subtest 6). Such a profile is, to say the least, extremely suspicious. The subject was a 25-year-old factory worker who was subsequently found to suffer from brain damage.

# INSTRUCTIONS FOR ADMINISTERING THE INTERVIEW

The material needed for the conduct of the interview is contained in the examination booklet which consists of the interview protocol, the items on which the interviewer is to record his judgments, special introductions, interviewer responses and probes.

At the outset, the interviewer should identify himself, offer to shake hands, and explain the purpose of the interview in a manner appropriate to the setting.

The interview protocol starts with a reference to the subject's opinions as the focus of interest, after which the interviewer asks the subject his name. The examiner should record the subject's name and an identification number on his answer sheet, the address or location where the interview is being conducted, his own name or code number, and the date. The interviewer should then proceed with the questions on date of birth, marital status, household composition, occupation, and schooling. The corresponding information should be recorded in the place provided at the top of the answer sheet. When follow-up interviews are conducted in close succession, the examiner, after the first couple of interviews, may omit the questions from date of birth through schooling, as they do not relate to specific items of the inventory. These questions have been segregated between dashed lines in the protocol.

## INTERVIEWER PROCEDURE

The interviewer should always present the stimuli in precisely the form shown in the protocol. Strict adherence to the interview protocol provides a standard stimulus situation which minimizes the effect of the interviewer's behavior on the subject and assures comparability across subjects. The procedure to be followed by the interviewer is analogous to that recommended for use in the administration of such psychological tests as the Wechsler Adult Intelligence Scale and the Stanford-Binet Scale. For the inventory to qualify as a standardized instrument, it is essential that the interviewer should not depart from the prescribed interview procedure.

If, at the beginning, the subject appears resistant or uneasy, the interviewer should seek to establish the necessary rapport before proceeding further. However, in order to maintain the standardized character of the interview, the interviewer should not expand the stimulus questions beyond the alternatives provided in the protocol.

In order to give a natural conversational quality to the interview as well as to make the stimuli fit the time and situation of the particular subject, a number of the stimuli are printed with an alternate word or phrase. The interviewer should choose the appropriate alternative expression. The alternatives are indicated either by a split line or by parentheses. If more than one of

41

the alternatives is appropriate, the interviewer should repeat the inquiry, substituting the other expression at the proper place. For example, at Question 93, if the subject is a recently admitted hospital patient the interviewer should ask first:

                    coworkers
"How are your neighbors treating you?"
                    classmates
Then, "How do the other patients treat you?"

But if the subject is a chronic resident patient, the first question will usually be omitted.

Before proceeding to the next stimulus, the interviewer should wait until he is quite sure that the subject has completed his answer. If the subject fails to respond to a specific question, the interviewer should wait quietly and with an air of expectancy for about half a minute to allow the silence to exercise some effect on the subject. Because mental patients are sometimes initially mute but warm up as the interview proceeds, the interviewer should in such cases return to the beginning of the protocol and repeat the questions up to the point where the subject began to respond, following the same order and tempo as in the initial presentation.

### Follow-up Questions

A limited number of follow-up stimuli have been provided in the protocol in parentheses to assure completeness of the subject's response. If the subject ignores or appears not to have heard one of the stimuli, the interviewer should repeat it in the same words. When the subject's response to a stimulus has been incomplete, the interviewer should use the parenthesized follow-up stimulus. Some examples follow:

    Q. "When is your birthday?"
    A. "May 27."
  (Q) "What year?"

    Q. "Tell me who lives(d) with you in your home."
    A. "I live alone."
  (Q) "What relatives do you have?"

(The choice of tense should always be contingent on the subject's circumstances. For example, in the above questions the choice hinges on whether the subject now lives in the community or in an institution.)

    Q. "What $\genfrac{}{}{0pt}{}{is}{was}$ your occupation?"

    A. "I $\genfrac{}{}{0pt}{}{am}{was}$ a secretary."

  (Q) "What $\genfrac{}{}{0pt}{}{do}{did}$ you do?"

Q. "Where do you work?"
A. "I used to work for the Redwood Lumber Company."
(Q) "Why did you stop?"
A. ". . ."
(Q) "What have you been doing since then?"

Q. "How far $\frac{\text{did you go}}{\text{are you}}$ in school?"
A. (Any level beyond elementary school.)
(Q) "What $\frac{\text{are}}{\text{were}}$ you studying?"

Q. "Tell me the date."
A. "It's the 10th."
(Q) "Month?", "Year?"

Q. "What is the name (address) of this place?"
(If the setting for the interview is an institution or a named public place, the interviewer should choose "name"; if the site is the subject's home or some other private location, then the interviewer should choose "address.")
A. "I don't remember the name."
(Q) "What kind of place is this?"

A. "It's a hospital."
(Q) "What kind of hospital?"

Q. "Where did you come from?"
A. "From the police station."
(Q) "Where were you before that?"

Q. "As you see it now, what was the reason that you came here?"
A. "I had taken some acid . . . and I was skipping down the street, ringing my bells, when I had a sudden impulse to take off my clothes . . . then this policeman chased me to my pad and brought me to the hospital."
(Q) "How do you feel about it now?"

Q. "What problems do you have?"
A. "I had to wash my hands so often that they got all raw . . . and I couldn't take care of the baby."
(Q) "What else can you tell me about your problems?"

Q. "What problems do you have?"
A. "Every time I have a few drinks I get into a fight."
(Q) "What are you doing about it?"

Q. "How is your mood today?"
A. "I don't know."
(Q) "What's your state of mind?"

Q. "What about your sense of humor?"
A. "Humor?" "What's humor?"
(Q) "What amuses you?"

Q. "Tell me about your family."
A. "Well, I have a mother and father, and there's my two sisters and a brother."
(Q) "How do you feel toward your family?"
A. "O.K."
(Q) "How do you feel about the way they treat(ed) you?"

Q. "Tell me about your social life."
A. "I don't go out much."
(Q) "What have you been doing together with other people?"

Q. "What have you been doing in your spare time?"
A. "Watching TV."
Q. "Tell me what interests you in the news."
A. "Haven't seen the paper."
Q. "What programs do you enjoy on TV or on the radio?"
A. "I just watch whatever is on."
(Q) "Tell me about your hobbies."

## Special Introductions

When an interview is repeated for purposes of short term follow-up, the interviewer should start by saying, "You might have answered some of these questions before, but I want to know how you feel about them now."

If a subject has anticipated any question in the protocol, the interviewer, when he reaches that question, should preface it with, "You (may) have answered this in part but. . . ." For example, if in response to the stimulus, "Tell me about your imagination," the subject mentions some of the things he thinks about, the interviewer should next say, "You have answered this in part, but what kinds of things have you been thinking about?"

If the subject's anticipatory answer was fairly complete and extensive, then instead of saying, "You've answered this in part, but . . .", the interviewer should say, "You've already told me about this, but I was going to ask you. . . ."

If the subject has anticipated a question just before the interviewer would have asked it in the normal sequence, the interviewer should not omit the question, but should preface it with: "I was just going to ask you. . . ."

44

The interview is intended to have a certain quality of ambiguity so as to force the subject himself to indicate by his choice what is important and significant for the assessment of current pathology. The interviewer should, therefore, avoid detailed or specific responses to the subject's request for clarification.

If the subject appears not to understand a particular question and asks what it means, the interviewer should repeat the question, placing emphasis on the important word in the question. He should not paraphrase it in his own words.

If the subject, in response to, "How is your mood today?" indicates that he doesn't understand the meaning of the word "mood," the interviewer should say, "What's your state of mind?"

If the subject asks for clarification as to the time referred to in a question, the interviewer should repeat the question emphasizing the present tense of the verb or repeat the question adding "now" to it. When the interviewer asks, "What is your health like?", if the subject replies by inquiring "Do you mean now or before I came here?", the interviewer should respond, "What is your health like in general?"

If the subject responds to the query, "What accidents have you had in which you hurt yourself?" by asking whether the interviewer means when he was a child or whether auto accidents are referred to, the interviewer should either indicate his acceptance of the first alternative by nodding or should reply, "Any."

If the subject, in response to the question, "What about your sense of humor?" indicates that he does not understand the meaning of the word "humor," the interviewer should say, "What amuses you?"

After the subject has responded to the question, "What about your sense of humor?" the interviewer should smile as he asks the next question. If the subject has smiled, the interviewer should stress the word, *"remember"*: "You still *remember* how to smile?" However, if the subject has not smiled up to this point, the interviewer should, nevertheless, smile himself, but should place the stress on the "smile": "You still remember how to *smile*?"

If in response to the inquiry, "Tell me about your family," the subject inquires whether the reference is to his parental or conjugal family, the interviewer should repeat the inquiry, substituting for "family" the person the subject offered first and, after the subject has finished what he has to say about the first family member, the interviewer should repeat the question, substituting the other family member as the focus of inquiry.

In response to "Tell me about your social life," or "What have you been doing in your spare time?", a recently hospitalized subject may ask, "Do

45

you mean now or before I came to the hospital?" In such cases the interviewer should respond with, "Recently."

The SCI is purposely designed so as to avoid invading the privacy of the subject. The subject's answer or refusal to answer a question or inquiry should be accepted by the interviewer without actual or implied criticism. This is in contrast to the procedure employed in a legal interrogation or in some judicial inquisitions. Moreover, except for the introductory questions about name, birthday, etc., the stimuli are for the most part of a general nature, intended to offer the subject an opportunity to express himself in his own way and to the extent that he is willing to disclose his feelings.

However, the stimuli are designed for the purpose of eliciting responses from which the interviewer can make the required judgments on the accompanying items. If the subject's reticence or hesitation leave the examiner uncertain as to the subject's meaning, he should attempt to resolve his uncertainty by using the soft probes provided as supplementary stimuli:

"Can you tell me (more) about $\begin{smallmatrix}\text{it}\\\text{that}\end{smallmatrix}$ ?"

"How much of a problem is $\begin{smallmatrix}\text{this}\\\text{it}\end{smallmatrix}$ for you (now)?"

"How do you feel about $\begin{smallmatrix}\text{this}\\\text{it}\\\text{that}\end{smallmatrix}$ (now)?"

"Why do you think that happens?"

The supplementary stimuli should be used as often as necessary to obtain completion of a response or to elicit additional data. But the interviewer should always keep in mind that the sole purpose of the interview is to provide responses from which he can answer the items. The interviewer should under no circumstances continue probing out of mere curiosity or to satisfy some clinical interest, as he might jeopardize the comparability of the case to the normative sample. Examples of appropriate use of a probe are:

Q. "As you see it now, what was the reason that you came here?"
A. "I had just gone to the apartment to get my clothes, but my husband called the police and they brought me here to the hospital."

Probe: "Can you tell me more about it?"

Q. "How is your memory?"

A. "It's not very good."

Probe: "How much of a problem is this for you?"

Q. "How about hurting yourself on purpose?"
A. "Last night, before I came here, I was so upset that I walked down the street and banged my fist against each parking meter as hard as I could."

Probe: "How do you feel about that now?"

Q. "What problems do you have?"
A. "I keep hearing his voice, but I don't see him."

Probe: "Why do you think that happens?"

### REINFORCEMENT

The interviewer should restrict his own reactions to such neutral responses as: "I see," "I understand," "Uh huh." These should always be uttered in a tone either of understanding or acceptance. In this way the interviewer will fulfill the minimal social requirements of the situation by reinforcing the subject for his communicativeness. The interviewer should carefully avoid any evaluative connotation in his response. If the subject asks for reassurance or information, the interviewer should parry such requests by expressing understanding or acceptance of the accompanying feeling and at the same time he should turn aside from the substantive content by indicating that he will return to it after completion of the interview or by indicating that it is outside his jurisdiction or competence, as the case may be.

### BEHAVIOR OF THE INTERVIEWER

The interviewer's task is a complex one. He must present the stimulus questions to the subject in a natural conversational tone with an air of professional interest, avoiding both too much detachment and too much sympathetic solicitude. He must respond to the subject with appropriate social grace but must not allow himself to become immersed in the subject's affect. At the same time, the interviewer, in his role as examiner, must be carefully observing the subject's expression and gestures and attending to the subtle cues of intonation, emphasis, choice of words, pauses, innuendoes; in short, to all the dimensions of communication which the experienced clinical interviewer relies on for making those first-order inferences that he is to record on the accompanying items.

Since the whole purpose of the interview is to obtain information for the judgments to be reported on the items, it behooves the interviewer to be thoroughly familiar with the items before he embarks on his first independent examination. He should have completed a training course under the guidance of an examiner experienced in this particular technique so as to resolve any ambiguities in the meanings of the items and so as to assure that his criteria of judgment conform with the standards by which the norms were established. In the course of training exercises or for the purpose of determining the reliability of inter-judge agreement, it may be desirable for two or even more examiners to participate in the examination. If two or more examiners are simultaneously present in the room with the subject, one of them should conduct the entire interview, while the others sit quietly alongside him observing and recording their judgments.

Although the interviewer would do well to learn the interview thoroughly before beginning his first interview, the examination booklet contains the interview protocol interspersed among the corresponding items. The interviewer is thus always provided with his next question and the items are located at those points where the relevant behavior or content is most likely to be elicited. The interviewer must not vary the order of his own lines, so as to preserve the standard quality of the structured interview, but he will need to range up and back among the items during the interview, adding or changing, as the case may require. The final statement, "Let me see if I have forgotten anything," is provided to give the interviewer an opportunity to make any necessary corrections or additions. In some circumstances, the interviewer may need to repeat an earlier question to verify a judgment or to obtain missing information. In such cases he should preface his question with "You may have answered this in part before, but. . . ."

## Marking the Items

The dichotomous inventory that accompanies the interview is the only formal record of the event that remains available for evaluation after the encounter. Although the whole encounter could be recorded on tape or even video, and such recordings of the interview have been found extremely useful for certain special studies and for training and demonstration purposes, it should be remembered that it takes just as long to replay an interview and to extract the relevant clinical data as it took to carry out the interview in the first instance. The 179 items which the examiner completes during the face-to-face encounter are the psychometric residue to be distilled out of the richness of the clinical confrontation. Like any distillate, they represent only a fraction of the live event. But it is precisely this fraction that is significant for the standardized comparisons of subjects with one another, with themselves before and after treatment, and with diagnostic groups. By always recording his judgments during the interview according to the same standards of judgment, the examiner maintains the essential psychometric qualify of his record.

The interviewer need not record the subject's verbatim responses, as the stimulus material has been devised specifically to evoke responses for the accompanying inventory. The interviewer should fill out the inventory as the interview is going on. The inventory should be finished before the subject leaves the room. This procedure insures that the information will be recorded while it is still fresh in mind and while any doubts or errors can be resolved.

The inventory is not concerned with background factors or case history. Behavior should therefore only be recorded either when it occurs at the time of the interview or when it is reported by the subject as a current feeling, attitude, or activity. For example, Item 29, "Says he gets irritablé or angry at the slightest provocation," requires that the subject tell substantially that this is a typical feature of his current behavior. However, this item does not include acting-out behavior during the course of the interview. Such behavior would be picked up by Item 148, "Loses his temper or has a fit of anger." In the same way, if the subject, in response to the questions about hurting himself, has reported that he made a suicidal attempt, the interviewer would have pursued this report with appropriate follow-up questions: "Can you tell me more about it?" "How much of a problem is this for you?" Only if he is satisfied that the subject still has thoughts about killing himself or still has a desire or intention to kill himself should the examiner record "Yes" for Item 59, "Indicates he is thinking about killing himself," or Item 60, "Indicates he wants or intends to kill himself." On the other hand, Item 61, "Reports that he deliberately does himself physical harm without intending his death," should be marked "Yes" if the subject describes this as a current attitude or disposition which has resulted in physical harm in the past and which is likely to occur again in the future.

Items that start with "Indicates," "Mentions," "Says," "Reports," require the observer to judge whether the subject has reported the substance of the content of the items. In order that the item be marked "Yes," it is not required that the subject must have expressed the pathology in precisely the words used in the item.

The subject may respond to a question by describing himself in general terms or by giving examples of the corresponding behavior. For example, Item 19, "Says that he is never upset or that nothing ever bothers him," requires a general statement from the subject, but Item 20, "Mentions that he worries a lot or that he cannot stop worrying," should be marked "Yes" if the subject actually describes himself this way, or if the subject, though not describing himself as a worrier, reports many instances of worrying behavior. Similarly, Item 32, "Describes himself as rash, impetuous, or impulsive," is marked "Yes" if the subject characterizes himself this way, but would also be marked "Yes" if the subject merely gives instances of this kind of behavior as typical of himself. With reference to depression, Item 17, "Reports that he has had more than one period of depression," should be marked "Yes" only if the subject reports recurrent depression, but not if he describes himself as depressed by one particular experience or loss. In the area of thought problems, Item 67, "Reports or expresses weird or bizarre thought," should be marked "Yes" if the subject qualifies his thoughts by these terms or similar terms, but also if he describes thoughts which are so patently absurd that the examiner can recognize them as weird or bizarre.

Item 2, "Perspires profusely or hand is wet or clammy," is best judged from a handshake at the beginning of the interview. Items 4 and 5 require reference to social norms for an appropriate judgment. Item 4, "Hair is unkempt, tangled or matted," should be marked "Yes" only if the hair is completely disheveled or dirty, but not if it is merely shaggy or cut in a bohemian style. Item 5, "Clothes are dirty, in disarray or bizarre," should only be marked "Yes" for instances of grossly incongruous combinations of clothing, dirty clothing not justified by work conditions, or transvestism.

For some items, even though it would be possible to secure corroboration, the interviewer should record his judgment on the basis of the evidence supplied by the subject. For example, Item 42, "Reports a motor or sensory dysfunction not confirmed by medical evidence," and Item 43, "Insists that an organ or organ system is diseased in spite of negative medical findings," refer to complaints by the subject about dysfunction or disease which are not supported by medical findings. The examiner should mark "Yes" for these items if the subject reports that his complaint has been rejected by medical authority or if he reports psychiatric referral as an ultimate consequence of a physical complaint. For Item 45, "Says that a part of his body is inexplicably changing in size or shape," to be marked "Yes," the subject has to make it clear that this change is mysterious to him.

### Criteria for Judgments

Answers to "Tell me about your imagination" vary from a noncommittal, "It's not very good," to a frank report of delusional or hallucinatory experiences. A noncommittal response may be belied by obvious indication of hallucinations. Significant behavior, both reported and observed, is recorded on the corresponding part of the inventory. The questions about social relations and about feelings toward the opposite sex commonly provoke verbal reports of problems. Often when no verbal report is forthcoming, increased movement, blushing, evasiveness, or observable discomfort make for a significant response.

In certain cases two or more items taken together reflect the dimension of intensity. For example, Item 107, "Mentions no plans for the future," together with Item 108, "Expresses a negative attitude toward his future accomplishments or attainments," provide a range of intensity for evaluating attitude toward the future. Only if the subject expresses complete absence of any planning for the future should Item 107 be rated "Yes." If he merely expresses a negative attitude, Item 108 should be rated "Yes" instead.

A few items refer to behavior which is only pathological if it occurs with some frequency during the interview. For example, Item 128, "Keeps talking about or coming back to some abstract topic (religion, politics, morals, etc.)," is marked "Yes" if the subject persistently reverts to some abstract topic. Similarly, Item 172, "Repeatedly laughs or giggles in a foolish way," and Item 173, "Repeatedly belches, clucks, grunts or grinds teeth," should not be marked "Yes" unless the corresponding behavior occurs over and over again. The examiner need not count the number of occasions but the behavior should occur with high frequency so that there is no question in his mind about its persistence.

Ambivalence should be distinguished from inconsistency. Thus Item 125, "Gives contradictory account of his experiences," should not be marked "Yes" merely because the subject expresses incompatible feelings toward some condition or event, but it should be marked "Yes" if his account is grossly inconsistent so that he has provided two competing explanations for either his behavior or his circumstances.

Inappropriate emotional response as reflected in Item 113, "Gives or reports incongruous emotional response (e.g., laughs or scoffs at occasion of death or disaster)," should be marked "Yes" only if the behavior is altogether out of keeping with the social implications of the event or condition. It should not be marked "Yes" merely because the subject laughs in embarrassment or smiles in recollection at his anger on some previous occasion.

Two components must be identified for Item 68, "Reports that a certain irrelevant thought intrudes on his consciousness," to be marked "Yes." The subject must refer to an intrusive thought, i.e., one which interferes with his train of thought, and it must seem irrelevant to him. If he is merely bothered by the occurrence of a certain thought, but that thought is not senseless, then this item should not be marked "Yes," but Item 66, "Reports that he broods over a certain unpleasant thought or feeling," should be marked "Yes" instead. On the other hand, if the subject reports the occurrence of a senseless thought but disclaims being bothered by it, then this is evidence for Item 67, "Reports or expresses weird or bizarre thought," but not for Item 66.

The area of interests is covered by a series of questions which seek to evoke from the subject some expression of what he likes to do on his own. If the subject, in response to the queries: "What have you been doing in your spare time?" "Tell me what interests you in the news," "What programs do you enjoy on TV or on the radio?" ("Tell me about your hobbies"), mentions something that currently interests him and that he likes to do, 104 and 105 are marked "No." Moreover, if the subject has at an earlier point in the interview indicated any present interest in work, school, family or social activities, or if he later expresses interest in planning for his future, he is marked "No" on Item 104. However, if he only mentions something that interests him or that he watches on TV or listens to on radio, but does not mention anything he likes to do or enjoys doing, then Item 105 should be marked "Yes." Thus, it is not enough for him to say that he watches or listens to program X on TV or radio; he has to indicate a current active enjoyment in watching or listening to the program to rate a "No" on Item 105.

Subjects vary in the amount of verbal output they display. Some subjects will speak extensively in response to each question and may even have to be interrupted by the interviewer in order that he may continue the interview. Other subjects are inclined to be laconic. They may answer rather briefly, but to the point. However, they may not elaborate their answers beyond the minimum response adequate to answer the questions. The examiner is not expected to distinguish between these two kinds of subjects. However, if the subject is so resistant that during the whole course of the interview he never does more than respond with single words or an occasional brief phrase, only then should Item 119, "Answers questions with single words or brief phrases only," be marked "Yes."

### SUPPLEMENTARY CRITERIA

Item 3. "Unshaven." If the subject *wears* a beard, do not mark "Yes."

Items 7–10. Mark "Yes" if the subject fails to provide the information for any reason, not only cognitive deficit, but resistiveness or secretiveness.

Item 12. "Circumstances." This refers to the specific conditions at the time when he moved into his house or came or was brought to a hospital or clinic. For example, Item 12 would be marked "Yes" whenever the subject either says or shows by his manner that he "Does not remember" that he moved here from another city or that he was brought to the hospital in an ambulance.

Item 13. Refers to the general conditions which provide a setting for his current status, his employment, his illness, his financial difficulty, etc. If the description of behavior is judged to be insufficient because the subject is either withholding information or is confabulating, then Item 13 and not Item 12 should be marked "Yes."

If the subject reports having been confused and not remembering the conditions under which he was hospitalized, 12 is marked "Yes" and 13 is marked "No," as the behavioral description is sufficient to account for his coming to the hospital.

If the subject is a patient, the interviewer must be satisfied that the behavior which precipitated admission is sufficiently described, even though the patient may not have insight. The patient may give enough of an account so that the interviewer recognizes the significance of the behavior. For example, the patient may have described an altercation with the manager of a store which resulted in the manager's calling the police. Although the patient said it wasn't justified, his description of his own belligerent behavior accounts for the subsequent admission.

Item 14. If the subject is a mental patient but denies his illness and blames someone else for his hospitalization; or if he admits illness, ascribing its cause to someone else, this item is marked "Yes."

Item 17. One of the depressions may be current.

Item 19. To qualify for a significant response the subject must express an attitude of *la belle indifference* and not merely indicate a lack of worry.

Item 21. "Keeps feeling afraid of different things" indicates a state in which the subject experiences feelings of fear in response to different stimuli in fairly rapid succession.

Item 30. "Drug addict," should include habituation to (but not occasional use of) nonaddictive drugs, e.g., hallucinogens (LSD, Mescaline, DMT, DET, STP) and marijuana, as well as addiction to amphetamines, barbiturates, or heroin.

Item 37. A patient who mentions having had a depression more than once is showing the behavior described in Item 17, but he shows that described in Item 37 only if he currently feels that way. For Item 37 the depression must be current not historical. (Use probe: "How do you feel about that now?")

Item 41. "Various aches and pains or physical dysfunctions" does not refer to a subject who reports a cold or headaches but to one who discusses a variety of vague and diffuse complaints that may or may not be true.

Items 49–52. Judge only with respect to current hallucination.

Item 59. In rating the behavior relating to Item 59 the examiner should judge very carefully whether a reference to a suicidal attempt in the past is purely historical or reflects some element of current attitude. If the examiner is uncertain he should be sure to add the standard follow-up question, "How much of a problem is this for you (now)?" Items 59, 60, 61 are marked "Yes" if the interviewer is satisfied that the subject, although referring to the past, still contemplates the activity as potential.

Item 63. The details forgotten must be important parts of the subject's own past experiences that he would be expected to remember (for example, his own birthday); otherwise dates are not important.

Item 66. For this item there must be some evidence of morbid preoccupation. If in doubt ask, "How much of a problem is it for you?"

Item 67. This item should be used to record an expression of thought which is completely out of context, grossly inappropriate, or downright inconsistent with nature.

Item 78. A subject should be considered to have "denounced" someone if he accuses him of a crime or of an unethical or immoral act; also, if he describes him as being uncouth or animal-like in his behavior.

Item 79. The subject need not use the word "hate" to qualify for a positive judgment on the examiner's part. An expression of strong dislike or distaste is sufficient. However, the examiner should be careful not to record a positive judgment if the subject merely indicates minor irritability or transient disagreement, making it clear that there is no deep hostility toward the other person.

Item 82. If the subject says that he avoids people, it is important to pursue with a follow-up question to see if he feels isolated. To identify this behavior the examiner must have the feeling tone from the subject.

Item 88. To qualify for a "Yes" on this item the subject must report or describe some habit or act which has occasioned difficulties with others, with authorities, or with the family.

Item 109. Of course, if the claim is actually impossible the observer should also mark the item "Yes."

Item 112. If the subject in general shows no gestural or facial movement, this qualifies him for a "Yes" on Item 171 rather than on Item 112. Moreover, if the subject, in describing a serious problem or encounter, indicates by his manner, attitude, or tone that he is controlling his own emotional response or that time or repetition have dulled his response, this would not qualify him for a "Yes" on Item 112. He must convey a mood of affectlessness, of lack of concern. On the other hand, if he displays affect which is in marked contrast to what is socially anticipated, then he gets "Yes" on Item 113 instead of Item 112.

Item 116. If at any point during the interview the subject asks whether the interviewer thinks he will regain some lost skill or ability, this is evidence for "Yes" on 116.

Item 120. This item should be used to reflect a cognitive difficulty in the subject's communication. It should not be used to record evasiveness or blocking or the kind of ambiguity that is premeditated because the subject doesn't want to disclose something he considers personal. The examiner should satisfy himself that he has the evidence for the above disturbance by employing the necessary follow-up question ("Can you tell me more about it?"). Item 120 calls for a judgment that the subject's discourse is private or ruminative rather than communicative or that he uses vague or symbolic language.

Item 128. The abstract topic could be completely irrelevant to the interview and the subject's circumstances, as, for example, if the subject keeps referring to some prominent political event.

# SCORING THE SCI

Since all the items are dichotomous and so worded that a mark of "Y" (YES) by the examiner indicates a judgment of psychopathology, the scorer need only concern himself with those items marked "Y." The scorer should first count the number of items for which the response, "Y," is checked in the examination booklet. This total should be entered in the corresponding box in the lower right-hand corner of the Scoring Sheet. He should next find and cross out on the Scoring Sheet the number corresponding to each of the items for which "Y" is checked in the examination booklet. He should then count the crossed-out numbers in each column (Subtest) of the Scoring Sheet and enter the sum in the appropriate box at the bottom. A check is performed by adding the subtest sums across the bottom to see if they agree with the total previously entered in the lower right-hand corner. Finally, the sum for each subtest should be transferred to the Profile Sheet on the line marked "Raw Score."

The raw scores should be converted to standard scores by reference to the Table of Standard Score Equivalents (Appendix A). The standard scores should be entered on the Profile Sheet on the line above the corresponding raw scores. To obtain a clinical profile, the standard scores should be plotted on the Profile Sheet and the successive points either connected by straight lines or circled for easier visualization. The ten standard scores should be added together and divided by ten to obtain the level (mean standard score) which should be represented by a bar in the column at the extreme left of the Profile Sheet.

# REFERENCES

Bartlett, M. S. The use of transformations. *Biometrics*, 1947, *3*, 39-52.

Burdock, E. I., Fleiss, J., & Hardesty, A. S. A new view of interobserver agreement. *Personnel Psychology*, 1963, *16*, 373-384.

Burdock, E. I., & Hardesty, A. S. Structured clinical interview and inventory. Paper presented at meeting of the Eastern Psychological Association, Atlantic City, N. J., 1962.

Burdock, E. I., & Hardesty, A. S. Behavior patterns of chronic schizophrenics. In P. H. Hoch & J. Zubin (Eds.), *Psychopathology of schizophrenia*. New York: Grune & Stratton, 1966. Pp. 182-204.

Burdock, E. I., & Hardesty, A. S. Psychological test for psychopathology. *Journal of Abnormal Psychology*, 1968, *73*, 62-69.

Burdock, E. I., & Hardesty, A. S. A research tactic for evaluation of drug specificity in schizophrenia. In D. V. Siva Sankar (Ed.), *Schizophrenia: Current Concepts and Research*. Hicksville, New York: P. J. D. Publications, 1969.

Burdock, E. I., & Hardesty, A. S. *Ward Behavior Inventory Manual*. New York: Springer, 1968.

Goldberg, S. C. & Mattsson, N. B. Schizophrenic subtypes defined by response to drugs and placebo. *Diseases of the Nervous System*, 1968, *29*, 153-158.

Landis, C. A. & Katz, S. E. The validity of certain measures which purport to measure neurotic tendencies. *Journal of Applied Psychology*, 1934, *18*, 343-356.

# APPENDIX A
Standard Score Equivalents for Raw Score Values
Adults and Adolescents

# APPENDIX B
Computer Program for Scoring SCI

# APPENDIX C
SCI Interview Booklet

# APPENDIX A    Standard Score Equivalents for Raw Score Values on the STRUCTURED CLINICAL INTERVIEW*    ADULTS

| Raw Score | 1 Anger-Hostility | 2 Conceptual Dysfunction | 3 Fear-Worry | 4 Incongruous Behavior | 5 Incongruous Ideation | 6 Lethargy-Dejection | 7** Perceptual Dysfunction | 8 Physical Complaints | 9 Self Depreciation | 10 Sexual Problems | Raw Score |
|---|---|---|---|---|---|---|---|---|---|---|---|
| 0 | -0.58 | -0.49 | -0.52 | -0.48 | -0.38 | -0.99 | 0 | -0.38 | -0.73 | -0.41 | 0 |
| 1 | 1.40 | 1.59 | 1.61 | 1.93 | 2.39 | 0.63 | 2.72 | 2.53 | 0.80 | 2.10 | 1 |
| 2 | 1.99 | 2.22 | 2.25 | 2.66 | 3.22 | 1.12 | 3.54 | 3.41 | 1.26 | 2.85 | 2 |
| 3 | 2.38 | 2.62 | 2.66 | 3.12 | 3.75 | 1.44 | 4.06 | 3.97 | 1.56 | 3.34 | 3 |
| 4 | 2.66 | 2.92 | 2.97 | 3.47 | 4.15 | 1.67 | 4.46 | 4.39 | 1.78 | 3.70 | 4 |
| 5 | 2.89 | 3.15 | 3.21 | 3.74 | 4.46 | 1.86 | 4.76 | 4.72 | 1.95 | 3.99 | 5 |
| 6 | 3.08 | 3.35 | 3.42 | 3.97 | 4.73 | 2.01 | 5.02 | 5.00 | 2.10 | 4.23 | 6 |
| 7 | 3.24 | 3.52 | 3.59 | 4.17 | 4.95 | 2.14 |  | 5.24 | 2.22 | 4.43 | 7 |
| 8 | 3.38 | 3.67 | 3.74 | 4.34 | 5.15 | 2.26 |  |  | 2.33 | 4.61 | 8 |
| 9 | 3.51 | 3.80 | 3.88 | 4.49 | 5.32 | 2.36 |  |  | 2.43 | 4.77 | 9 |
| 10 | 3.62 | 3.92 | 4.00 | 4.63 | 5.48 | 2.45 |  |  | 2.52 |  | 10 |
| 11 | 3.72 | 4.02 | 4.11 | 4.75 | 5.62 | 2.54 |  |  | 2.60 |  | 11 |
| 12 | 3.82 | 4.12 | 4.21 | 4.87 | 5.75 | 2.61 |  |  | 2.67 |  | 12 |
| 13 | 3.90 | 4.21 |  | 4.97 | 5.87 | 2.68 |  |  | 2.74 |  | 13 |
| 14 | 3.98 | 4.30 |  | 5.07 | 5.99 | 2.75 |  |  | 2.80 |  | 14 |
| 15 | 4.06 | 4.38 |  | 5.16 | 6.09 | 2.81 |  |  | 2.86 |  | 15 |
| 16 | 4.13 | 4.45 |  | 5.25 | 6.19 | 2.87 |  |  | 2.91 |  | 16 |
| 17 | 4.19 | 4.52 |  | 5.33 | 6.28 | 2.92 |  |  | 2.96 |  | 17 |
| 18 | 4.26 | 4.58 |  | 5.40 | 6.37 |  |  |  | 3.01 |  | 18 |
| 19 | 4.32 | 4.65 |  | 5.48 | 6.45 |  |  |  | 3.05 |  | 19 |
| 20 | 4.37 | 4.71 |  | 5.54 | 6.53 |  |  |  | 3.10 |  | 20 |
| 21 | 4.43 | 4.76 |  | 5.61 | 6.60 |  |  |  |  |  | 21 |
| 22 | 4.48 | 4.82 |  | 5.67 | 6.68 |  |  |  |  |  | 22 |
| 23 | 4.53 | 4.87 |  | 5.73 | 6.74 |  |  |  |  |  | 23 |
| 24 | 4.57 | 4.92 |  | 5.79 | 6.81 |  |  |  |  |  | 24 |
| 25 | 4.62 | 4.96 |  | 5.84 | 6.87 |  |  |  |  |  | 25 |
| 26 | 4.66 | 5.01 |  |  | 6.93 |  |  |  |  |  | 26 |
| 27 | 4.70 | 5.05 |  |  | 6.99 |  |  |  |  |  | 27 |
| 28 |  | 5.09 |  |  | 7.04 |  |  |  |  |  | 28 |

To obtain Level add standard scores of 10 subtests and divide by 10.

*Based on reference population of 95 normals.

**Based on 183 mental patients because all normals scored zero.

12/7/66

58

## Standard Score Equivalents for Raw Score Values on the STRUCTURED CLINICAL INTERVIEW*

| Raw Score | 1 Anger-Hostility | 2 Conceptual Dysfunction | 3 Fear-Worry | 4 Incongruous Behavior | 5** Incongruous Ideation | 6 Lethargy-Dejection | 7*** Perceptual Dysfunction | 8 Physical Complaints | 9 Self Depreciation | 10 Sexual Problems | Raw Score |
|---|---|---|---|---|---|---|---|---|---|---|---|
| 0 | -0.43 | -0.46 | -0.40 | -0.25 | -0.38 | -0.73 | 0 | -0.25 | -0.39 | -0.30 | 0 |
| 1 | 1.67 | 1.69 | 2.20 | 3.47 | 2.39 | 0.96 | 2.72 | 3.88 | 1.75 | 3.32 | 1 |
| 2 | 2.30 | 2.34 | 2.99 | 4.59 | 3.22 | 1.47 | 3.54 | 5.12 | 2.39 | 4.41 | 2 |
| 3 | 2.70 | 2.75 | 3.49 | 5.31 | 3.75 | 1.79 | 4.06 | 5.92 | 2.80 | 5.11 | 3 |
| 4 | 3.00 | 3.06 | 3.86 | 5.84 | 4.15 | 2.04 | 4.46 | 6.51 | 3.11 | 5.63 | 4 |
| 5 | 3.24 | 3.31 | 4.16 | 6.27 | 4.46 | 2.23 | 4.76 | 6.98 | 3.36 | 6.04 | 5 |
| 6 | 3.44 | 3.51 | 4.41 | 6.62 | 4.73 | 2.39 | 5.02 | 7.37 | 3.56 | 6.38 | 6 |
| 7 | 3.61 | 3.69 | 4.62 | 6.92 | 4.95 | 2.53 | | | 3.73 | 6.68 | 7 |
| 8 | 3.76 | 3.84 | 4.81 | 7.19 | 5.15 | 2.65 | | | 3.89 | 6.93 | 8 |
| 9 | 3.89 | 3.98 | 4.97 | 7.42 | 5.32 | 2.76 | | | 4.02 | 7.16 | 9 |
| 10 | 4.01 | 4.10 | 5.12 | 7.64 | 5.48 | 2.85 | | | 4.14 | | 10 |
| 11 | 4.12 | 4.21 | 5.25 | 7.83 | 5.62 | 2.94 | | | 4.25 | | 11 |
| 12 | 4.22 | 4.31 | 5.38 | 8.00 | 5.75 | 3.02 | | | 4.36 | | 12 |
| 13 | 4.31 | 4.41 | | 8.17 | 5.87 | 3.09 | | | 4.45 | | 13 |
| 14 | 4.40 | 4.49 | | 8.32 | 5.99 | 3.16 | | | 4.54 | | 14 |
| 15 | 4.48 | 4.58 | | 8.46 | 6.09 | 3.23 | | | 4.62 | | 15 |
| 16 | 4.55 | 4.65 | | 8.59 | 6.19 | 3.29 | | | 4.69 | | 16 |
| 17 | 4.62 | 4.72 | | 8.71 | 6.28 | 3.34 | | | 4.76 | | 17 |
| 18 | 4.69 | 4.79 | | 8.83 | 6.37 | | | | 4.83 | | |
| 19 | 4.75 | 4.86 | | 8.94 | 6.45 | | | | 4.90 | | |
| 20 | 4.81 | 4.92 | | 9.05 | 6.53 | | | | 4.96 | | |
| 21 | 4.86 | 4.97 | | 9.15 | 6.60 | | | | | | |
| 22 | 4.92 | 5.03 | | 9.24 | 6.68 | | | | | | |
| 23 | 4.97 | 5.08 | | 9.34 | 6.74 | | | | | | |
| 24 | 5.02 | 5.13 | | 9.42 | 6.81 | | | | | | |
| 25 | 5.07 | 5.18 | | 9.51 | 6.87 | | | | | | |
| 26 | 5.11 | 5.23 | | | 6.93 | | | | | | |
| 27 | 5.16 | 5.27 | | | 6.99 | | | | | | |
| 28 | | 5.32 | | | 7.04 | | | | | | |

To obtain level add standard scores of 10 subtests and divide by 10.

*Based on 49 normal adolescents 16–17 years of age.

**Based on 95 normal adults because all adolescents scored zero.

***Based on 183 mental patients because all normals scored zero.

### Fortran IV Computer Program for scoring SCI from item responses

```
C     THIS SCI SCORE PROGRAM SCORES ITEMS DIRECTLY FROM THE SCI ANSWER
C     SHEETS. IT YIELDS RAW, TRANSFORMED AND STANDARD SCORES FOR EACH
C     OF THE SUBTESTS AND FOR LEVEL.
C     INPUT CONSIST OF
C        CARD 1 COL 1- 3  ITMNO = NO. OF ITEMS FOR EACH SUBJECT = 179
C                      4  KARD  = NO OF CARDS NEEDED            = 4
C                    5- 6  IAREA = NO. OF SUBTESTS FOR SCI      = 10
C                    7-10  N     = NO. OF SUBJECTS
C        CARDS 2-4    IAS(I) =ASSIGNMENT OF ITEMS TO SUBTESTS [a]
C        CARDS 5-   ITEM CARDS BEGIN. ITEM CARDS CONTAIN 2 SECTIONS
C           SECTION 1 COLS 1-29 IDEN = IDENTIFICATION - CONTAINS
C                         1 = KARNO = CARD NO
C                       2-5 = KODSTY= STUDY CODE
C                      6-15 = IDSUBJ= SUBJECT ID
C                     16-19 = LOCOD = LOCATION CODE
C                     20-23 = INTCOD= INTERVIEWER CODE
C                     24-29 = IDATE = DATE OF INTERVIEW
C                     30-35 = BLANKS
C           SECTION 2  36-80 = ITEMS = ITEMS 1-45/CARD 1, 46-90/CARD2
C                                  91-135/CARD 3 136-179/CARD4
C     OUTPUT CONTAIN
C        1. RAW SCORES
C        2. TRANSFORMED SCORES
C        3. STANDARD SCORES
C
      DIMENSION ICARD(80), IDEN(29), ITEM(179), IAS(179), R (10),
     1 T (10), S (10), TM(10), TST(10)
      REAL TM/0.2596, 0.2064, 0.2161, 0.1744, 0.1197, 0.5370, 0.0000,
     1 0.1141, 0.4200, 0.1438/, TST/0.4445, 0.4243, 0.4133, 0.3660,
     2 0.3191, 0.5429, 0.3242, 0.3029, 0.5756, 0.3512/
      REAL LEVELS
      EQUIVALENCE (ICARD, IDEN)
      NPAGE = 1
      READ 2, ITMNO, KARD, IAREA, N
    2 FORMAT(I3, I1, I2, I4)
      READ 3,(IAS(I), I=1,179)
    3 FORMAT(80I1)
      EN = N
      M = IAREA
      CASES = EN
   20 PRINT 1, NPAGE
    1 FORMAT('1', 45X, 'SCI SCORE PROGRAM', 45X, 'PAGE', 2X, I2)
      PRINT 21
   21 FORMAT('0', 70X, 'SUBTESTS',//, 58X, '1', 5X, '2', 5X, '3', 5X,
     1 '4', 5X, '5', 5X, '6', 5X, '7', 5X, '8', 5X, '9', 5X, '10', 2X,
     2 'LEVEL',//)
      NPAGE = NPAGE + 1
      LINES = 0
    4 J = 1
    5 READ 3, (ICARD(L), L=1,80)
      DO 6 K=36,80
      ITEM(J) = ICARD(K)
      IF(J.EQ.179)GO TO 100
    6 J=J+1
      GO TO 5
  100 DO 10 I=1,10
   10 R (I) = 0.0
      DO 11 I=1,ITMNO
      IF(IAS(I).EQ.0)IAS(I) = 10
      INDEX = IAS(I)
   11 R (INDEX) = R (INDEX) + ITEM(I)
C     RAW SCORES ARE OBTAINED
      DO 12 I=1,M
   12 T (I) = ALOG(SQRT(R (I)) + SQRT(R (I) + 1.0))
C     TRANSFORMED SCORES ARE OBTAINED
      DO 13 I=1,M
      S (I) = (T (I) - TM(I)) / TST(I)
   13 CONTINUE
      SSUM = 0.0
      DO 24 I=1,M
      SSUM = SSUM + S(I)
   24 CONTINUE
      LEVELS = SSUM/10.0
C     STANDARD SCORES ARE OBTAINED
      PRINT 15, (IDEN(I), I=1,29), (R (I), I=1,M)
   15 FORMAT('0RAW SCORES', 10X, 29I1, 5X, 10F6.2)
      PRINT 16, (IDEN(I), I=1,29), (T (I), I=1,M)
   16 FORMAT(' TRANSFORMED SCORES', 2X, 29I1, 5X, 10F6.2)
      PRINT 17, (IDEN(I), I=1,29), (S (I), I=1,M), LEVELS
   17 FORMAT(' STANDARD SCORES', 5X, 29I1, 5X, 11F6.2)
      CASES = CASES - 1.0
      IF (CASES) 14,14,50
   50 LINES = LINES + 2
      IF (LINES - 20) 4, 20, 4
   14 CALL EXIT
      END
```

B. W.          APRIL, 1969          BIOMETRIC LAB, NYU MEDICAL CENTER

# APPENDIX C

## Structured Clinical Interview

"I want to get your personal opinions about your situation."

1. Shuffles or drags feet .................................................. Y  N

2. Perspires profusely or hand is wet or clammy ......................... Y  N

3. Face is dirty or unshaven............................................. Y  N

4. Hair is unkempt, tangled or matted.................................... Y  N

5. Clothes are dirty, in disarray or bizarre............................ Y  N

6. Smells of urine or feces............................................. Y  N

"First, spell your name for me, please."

7. Fails to give his name............................................... Y  N

------------------------------------------------

"What is your date of birth?" ("What year?")
"Are you married or single?"
"Tell me who lives(d) with you in your home."

("Who else $\frac{is}{was}$ in the household?")

("What relatives do you have?")

"What $\frac{is}{was}$ your occupation?" ("What $\frac{do}{did}$ you do?")

"Where $\frac{do}{did}$ you $\frac{work}{go\ to\ school}$?" ("Why did you stop?")

("What have you been doing since then?")

"How far $\frac{did\ you\ go}{are\ you}$ in school?"

("What $\frac{are}{were}$ you studying?")

------------------------------------------------

"What is the date today?" ("month?", "year?")

8. Fails to specify month and year......................................... Y  N

"What is the name (address) of this place?"

9. Fails to mention institution or street................................. Y  N

("What kind of place is this?")
("What kind of hospital?")

10. Fails to identify the general nature of his
surroundings (hospital, home, clinic, etc.)............................. Y  N

"How long have you been here?"
"Where did you come from?"
("Where were you before that?")
"As you see it now, what was the reason that you came here?"
("How do you feel about it now?")

11. Assumes incorrect role (e.g., says he is here as a
visitor, worker or staff member)...........................................Y  N

12. Does not remember the circumstances under which
he came to home, hospital or clinic................................... Y  N

13. Gives a description of his behavior which is implausible
or insufficient to account for his present situation (e.g.,
is unable to tell what he does or has been doing)...........Y  N

14. Places entire responsibility for his illness, situation
or hospitalization on someone else................................. Y  N

"What problems do you have?"

15. Mentions that he is bothered by feeling of
nervousness or anxiety.............................................. Y  N

16. Tells about a period of elation.................................... Y  N

17. Reports that he has had more than one period of
depression......................................................... Y  N

18. Says he feels nothing, has no feelings or his
feelings have dried up............................................. Y  N

19. Says that he is never upset or that nothing ever
bothers him........................................................ Y  N

20. Mentions that he worries a lot or that he cannot
stop worrying...................................................... Y  N

("What else can you tell me about your problems?")

("What are you doing about $\frac{it}{your\ problems}$?")

21. Mentions that he has lots of fears or that he keeps
feeling afraid of different things................................. Y  N

22. Indicates a fear of going insane, having a nervous
breakdown, or losing control of his emotions................ Y  N

23. Indicates that he has an irrational fear of a particular
object or situation (e.g., crowds, heights).................. Y  N

24. Speaks of concern about attack of panic.................... Y  N

25. Describes a fit of violent rage.......................... Y  N

26. Mentions some act or routine which he repeats
excessively and which he cannot resist repeating
(e.g., washing hands, checking locks, etc.).............. Y  N

27. Indicates that he has more than once been in
trouble with the law............................................. Y  N

28. Reports act of cruelty, violence or arson with
obvious enjoyment................................................ Y  N

29. Says he gets irritable or angry at the slightest
provocation........................................................ Y  N

30. Indicates that he is an alcoholic or drug addict............. Y  N

31. Says that someone is in his mind or body or that
he is "possessed" by a spirit or devil......................... Y  N

32. Describes himself as rash, impetuous or impulsive ................. Y  N

33. Says that he cannot make up his mind or that he has difficulty making decisions............................. Y  N

34. Indicates that he thinks about committing or feels he might commit some horrible act (e.g., that he might attack or kill someone).................................... Y  N

35. Indicates that he enjoys thinking about tragic or horrible events............................................ Y  N

"How is your mood today?"  ("What's your state of mind?")

36. Indicates that he feels elated or high........................................ Y  N

37. Mentions that he feels depressed or despondent....................... Y  N

38. Mentions that he feels he is getting nowhere,........................... Y  N

"What is your health like?"

39. Indicates that he has trouble sleeping or that he requires drugs to sleep........................... Y  N

"How do you feel today?"

40. Indicates that he feels tired, sleepy or without energy.......... Y  N

41. Mentions that he has various aches and pains or physical dysfunctions................................. Y  N

42. Reports a motor or sensory dysfunction not confirmed by medical evidence............................ Y  N

43. Insists that an organ or organ system is diseased in spite of negative medical findings........................... Y  N

44. Expresses dissatisfaction with his size or strength.................. Y  N

45. Says that a part of his body is inexplicably changing in size or shape................................. Y  N

46. Says that his body is decaying or rotting............................ Y  N

47. Imagines that he has a fatal illness or that he is about to die.. Y  N

48. Expresses dissatisfaction with the appearance of his body or part of his body...................................... Y  N

"How is your eyesight?"
"What happens when you close your eyes?"

49. Indicates that he experiences visual perceptions in the absence of an adequate or appropriate stimulus...................... Y  N

50. Indicates that objects or people look unusually large or small........................................ Y  N

51. Indicates that people or things look weird or distorted.......... Y  N

"How is your hearing?"

52. Indicates that he experiences auditory perceptions in the absence of an adequate or appropriate stimulus..................... Y  N

53. Says that he gets creeping or crawling sensation on his body.. Y  N

"How does your head feel?"

54. Speaks of attack of palpitations, faintness, dizziness or unsteadiness...................................... Y  N

"How do you enjoy eating?"

55. Says that he has lost his appetite or the capacity to enjoy food.......................................... Y  N

("How does your food taste to you?")

56. Reports that his food tastes or looks suspicious or that he is being poisoned...................... Y  N

"How is your sense of smell?"

57. Indicates that he notices smells in the absence of an adequate or appropriate stimulus........................... Y  N

58. Claims that he just has a physical ailment in spite of evidence of psychological disturbance........................ Y  N

"What accidents have you had in which you hurt yourself?"
"What have you done that's dangerous?"
"How about hurting yourself on purpose?"

59. Indicates he is thinking about killing himself..................... Y  N

60. Indicates he wants or intends to kill himself...................... Y  N

61. Reports that he deliberately does himself physical harm without intending his death........................ Y  N

"How is your memory?"

62. Mentions that his memory is impaired or that he keeps forgetting things................................ Y  N

63. Reports difficulty in recalling important details of past experience.................................. Y  N

64. Tells of fit, seizure or lapse of consciousness................... Y  N

"Tell me about your imagination."

65. Reports that he engages in wishful thinking instead of working................................ Y  N

"What kinds of things have you been thinking about?"

66. Reports that he broods over a certain unpleasant thought or feeling................................ Y  N

67. Reports or expresses weird or bizarre thought.................. Y  N

68. Reports that a certain irrelevant thought intrudes on his consciousness.................................. Y  N

69. Reports that things seem unreal or dreamlike..................... Y  N

70. Says that he feels as if he is outside of his body, or as if his body does not belong to him........................... Y  N

"What about your sense of humor?"
("What amuses you?")

71. Says he has lost his sense of humor............................... Y  N

"You still remember how to smile?"

72. Does not smile either spontaneously or in response to suggestion........................................ Y  N

"Tell me about your family."
                          husband
                          wife
("Tell me about your  parents." )
                          father
                          mother

                          him
("How do you feel toward her      ?")
                          your family

73. Says that he is unwilling to see any member of his immediate family........................................ Y  N

# Structured Clinical Interview

74. Expresses jealousy, rivalry or bitter envy ........................... Y  N

75. Says he does not care what happens to his family.................. Y  N

("How do you feel about the way she he treat(s) you?")
("How do you feel about the way they treated you?")

76. Tells how his family has mistreated or harmed him................. Y  N

77. Expresses a desire to harm relative, friend or associate........... Y  N

78. Denounces relative, friend or associate.................................. Y  N

79. Expresses hatred for relative, acquaintance or associate.......... Y  N

"Tell me about your social life."
("What have you been doing together with other people?")

80. Says people avoid, reject or dislike him ............................... Y  N

81. Mentions that he feels inhibited or uncomfortable with people....................................................................... Y  N

82. Mentions that he feels distant or isolated from people........... Y  N

"What friends do you have now?"

83. Reports that he has no friends or that he cannot make or keep friends......................................................................... Y  N

84. Says that there is no one he can talk to or confide in............. Y  N

"How do you feel toward the opposite sex?"

"How do you feel toward other men ?"
"How do you feel toward other women ?"

85. Becomes flustered when asked about his relations with the opposite sex or expresses feeling of fear or discomfort..... Y  N

86. Says that he has difficulty getting along with the opposite sex............................................................................... Y  N

87. Reports that he is impotent, frigid or deficient in sexual performance......................................................................... Y  N

88. Reports that he has more than once been in trouble because of his sexual habits..................................................... Y  N

89. Indicates that he feels troubled about masturbation............... Y  N

90. Reports sexual practice or desire which is different from that of most people (e.g., homosexuality, nyphomania, etc.)........ Y  N

91. Indicates that he feels he is being punished for his sin or immorality............................................................................. Y  N

92. Expresses feeling of guilt............................................................. Y  N

"How are your coworkers / your neighbors / your classmates / the other patients treating you?"

93. Reports that he gets angry when criticized............................ Y  N

94. Tells how peer or stranger has mistreated or harmed him...... Y  N

95. Says that person in position of authority or power has mistreated or harmed him (e.g., staff member, policeman, employer, etc.).............................................. Y  N

96. Mentions that people take advantage of him or push him around.......................................................................... Y  N

97. Says he does not care how his behavior harms other people............................................................................... Y  N

98. Indicates that he detects a personal reference in seemingly insignificant remark or event.................................. Y  N

99. Says that someone talks about him or ridicules him...................................................................................... Y  N

100. Expresses a belief that he has been harassed or persecuted which is almost certainly not true (e.g., he has been followed by members of a secret organization)............................................................................ Y  N

101. Mentions that he hits or attacks people or some person........................................................................................ Y  N

102. Claims that his mind or actions are controlled or mysteriously influenced by other person or by strange force....................................................................... Y  N

103. Indicates a belief that someone wants to hurt him.......... Y  N

"What have you been doing in your spare time?"
"Tell me what interests you in the news."
"What programs do you enjoy on TV or on the radio?"
("Tell me about your hobbies.")

104. Mentions nothing that interests him................................ Y  N

105. Mentions nothing that he enjoys doing............................ Y  N

106. Expresses feeling of inferiority or inadequacy.................. Y  N

"What plans are you making for the future?"

107. Mentions no plans for the future...................................... Y  N

108. Expresses a negative attitude toward his future accomplishments or attainments.................................... Y  N

109. Speaks of contact, power, knowledge or sensational plan which though not impossible is extremely unlikely (e.g., says the President will come to take him out of the hospital).................................................. Y  N

110. Indicates that he does not recognize that his behavior is evidence of a psychological disturbance...................... Y  N

"How do you feel about the way things are going for you?"

111. Expresses intense regret for something he has done or failed to do................................................................ Y  N

112. Talks of a serious personal problem in a flat unemotional manner........................................................... Y  N

113. Gives or reports incongruous emotional response (e.g., laughs or scoffs at occasion of death or disaster)....... Y  N

"How do you feel about talking to me today?"

114. Expresses resentment about one of the questions.............. Y  N

115. Accuses interviewer of misrepresentation......................... Y  N

116. Presses for help or reassurance......................................... Y  N

117. Misidentifies the role of the interviewer (e.g., refers to interviewer as relative, patient, guard, etc.).................. Y  N

118. Acts contemptuous or insulting (e.g., sarcastically mispronounces interviewer's name, challenges interviewer's competence, etc.)......................................................... Y  N

"What else should I ask you?"

119. Answers questions with single words or brief phrases only....................................................................................... Y  N

120. Makes explanation in an ambiguous, obscure or cryptic manner................................................................ Y N

121. Repeats word or phrase in a mechanical manner (e.g., ("Please be so kind, please be so kind.")...................... Y N

122. Mixes up words, makes up new words or talks gibberish........ Y N

123. Talks in an aimless and digressive fashion......................... Y N

124. Adds minute details or makes elaborate qualifications........... Y N

125. Gives contradictory account of his experiences..................... Y N

126. Assumes the identity of a famous figure or makes impossible claim of personal fame (e.g., "The whole country knows me," "I am Mary, Mother of God")............Y N

127. Claims power or knowledge beyond the bounds of credibility (e.g., gets personal messages from God, can read minds, has solution to mankind's ills)..................... Y N

128. Keeps talking about or coming back to some abstract topic (religion, politics, morals, etc.)............................ Y N

129. Forgets what he is talking about...................................... Y N

130. More than once shifts attention to unimportant object or incidental sound......................................................... Y N

131. Becomes preoccupied or shows lapse of attention................. Y N

132. Talks on and on and resists interruption........................... Y N

133. Talks to himself........................................................... Y N

134. Speaks in a faint voice or voice becomes weak or fades away............................................................................ Y N

135. Speaks belligerently..................................................... Y N

136. Shouts and yells or curses and swears.............................. Y N

137. Pitch of voice shows no variation (i.e., completely monotonous)................................................................. Y N

"Let me see if I have forgotten anything."

138. Speaks extremely rapidly and with infrequent pauses........... Y N

139. Speech is both slow and full of pauses............................. Y N

140. Speech is blurred or inarticulate.................................... Y N

141. Stutters or stammers.................................................... Y N

142. Speech is at times inaudible or incoherent......................... Y N

143. Makes menacing gesture or physical attack......................... Y N

144. Throws something.......................................................... Y N

145. Bangs fist on table or stamps foot.................................. Y N

146. Deliberately tears or breaks something.............................. Y N

147. Continually looks angry.................................................. Y N

148. Loses his temper or has a fit of anger.............................. Y N

149. Gesticulates excitedly................................................... Y N

150. Is overcome by frenzied excitement................................... Y N

151. Shows fleeting and rapidly alternating facial expressions........ Y N

152. Expresses feeling of extravagant elation............................ Y N

153. Has a sad expression or holds his body in a dejected or despondent posture.................................................Y N

154. Sighs repeatedly.......................................................... Y N

155. Weeps, moans or wrings hands........................................ Y N

156. Has a frightened or apprehensive expression........................Y N

157. Has attack of panicky fear............................................. Y N

158. Remains immobile throughout the interview........................ Y N

159. Turns away, turns his back, gets up from his seat or tries to leave room.................................................. Y N

160. Stands up throughout the interview.................................. Y N

161. Continually rubs, scratches or licks himself or pulls out hair or picks at skin............................................... Y N

162. Keeps eyes closed or head averted throughout the interview..................................................................... Y N

163. Grasps, pulls or tugs limbs or clothing............................. Y N

164. Ceremoniously performs some apparently irrelevant act........ Y N

165. Writhes or contorts body............................................... Y N

166. Gets up and moves about restlessly.................................. Y N

167. Plays with or exposes genitals........................................ Y N

168. Assumes strange pose for no apparent reason...................... Y N

169. Has tic or twitch (e.g., distorts face, turns neck, blinks)......... Y N

170. Fidgets or squirms in his seat........................................ Y N

171. Maintains impassive expression except for brief interruption.................................................................. Y N

172. Repeatedly laughs or giggles in a foolish way.................... Y N

173. Repeatedly belches, clucks, grunts or grinds teeth................. Y N

174. Has tremor of hand or fingers........................................ Y N

175. Is slow in all his movements........................................... Y N

176. Makes sexual suggestion................................................ Y N

177. Makes overt sexual advance (e.g., caress).......................... Y N

178. Shows difficulty recalling recent events............................. Y N

179. Says only a few words or does not talk at all...................... Y N

64